Cardiac Arrhythmias: Self-Assessment

Volume 2

Cardiac Arrhythmias: Self-Assessment

Volume 2

Edward K. Chung
M.D., F.A.C.P., F.A.C.C.

Professor of Medicine
Jefferson Medical College of
Thomas Jefferson University and
Director of the Heart Station and
Attending Physician (Cardiologist)
Thomas Jefferson University Hospital
Philadelphia, PA. 19107

Fellow, American College of Cardiology
Former Governor for West Virginia, American College of Cardiology
Fellow, American College of Physicians
Member, American Federation for Clinical Research
Member, American Heart Association
Member, American Medical Association

Editorial Board Member for *Cardiology,*
The Journal of Electrocardiology, Heart and
Lung, Drug Therapy, Primary Cardiology,
and *Hospital Physician*

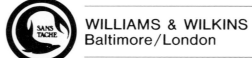

WILLIAMS & WILKINS
Baltimore/London

Volume One 1977
Reprinted January 1979
Reprinted October 1979

Other books by Dr. Chung include:
Digitalis Intoxication, 1970.
Principles of Cardiac Arrhythmias, Second Edition, 1977.
Cardiac Arrhythmias: Self Assessment, Volume—I, 1977.
Artificial Cardiac Pacing: Practical Approach, 1979.
Exercise Electrocardiography: Practical Approach, 1979.

Library of Congress Cataloging in Publication Data

Chung, Edward K.
    Cardiac arrhythmias.
    Bibliography: v. 1. p.
    Includes indexes.
    1. Arrhythmia—Diagnosis. 2. Electrocardiography. I. Title [DNLM: 1. Arrhythmia—Diagnosis—Examination questions. 2. Electrocardiography—Atlases. WG 18 C559c 1977]
RC685.A65C47   616.1′280754   77-4111
ISBN 0-683-01574-5 (v. 2)   AACR2

Composed and printed at the
Waverly Press, Inc.
Mt. Royal and Guilford Aves.
Baltimore, Md. 21202, U.S.A.

To My Wife, Lisa
and
To My Children,
Linda and Christopher

Preface

Since 1977, when the first volume of this book was published, extensive studies have been carried out in the fields of the sick sinus syndrome and bradytachyarrhythmia syndrome, bifascicular block and trifascicular block, and artificial cardiac pacing. Thus, a new chapter on the sick sinus syndrome and bradytachyarrhythmia syndrome is added, and the chapters dealing with artificial cardiac pacing and various intraventricular conduction disturbances have been significantly expanded. In addition, in-depth discussion regarding differential diagnosis of various cardiac arrhythmias is included in this book because it is probably the most important, yet the most difficult, problem which every physician will confront in daily practice.

Volume II presents 200 electrocardiographic tracings, with a short case history for each to aid in the interpretation of the electrocardiogram. The reverse side of each page gives a full analysis of the interpretation of the tracing so that the reader can assess his/her diagnosis. In the majority of cases, 3 simultaneous leads (leads V_1, II, and V_5) recorded by 3-channel ECG equipment, are shown for the accurate diagnosis. In addition to the electrocardiographic diagnosis, the pertinent clinical significance and the therapeutic approach are included in many instances. The primary intention of the author is to describe common cardiac arrhythmias which are frequently encountered in daily practice.

The arrangement of the text and illustrations is based upon the author's experience in teaching medical students, house staff, cardiology fellows, cardiac care nurses, and primary physicians with various backgrounds. This volume is intended as a companion to the first volume (published in 1977) as well as to the traditional textbook entitled, *Principles of Cardiac Arrhythmias*, Third Edition, published recently by the same publisher, Williams & Wilkins. Thanks to many readers, as well as to the reviewers, these books have been well received.

The unique feature of Volume II, like all other books by the author, is a practical approach with its clinical applications which will directly assist each reader in the diagnosis and management of his/her patient. The author hopes that the book will be of a particular value to all **vii** primary physicians including cardiologists, internists, family physicians, and emergency room physicians, in addition to medical house staff and cardiology fellows. Medical students, cardiac care nurses, and physicians with other specialities (e.g., anesthesiologists), of course, will learn about various cardiac arrhythmias in detail by reading this book.

The secretarial burden was carried out cheerfully by Miss Veronica Sevick, personal secretary to the author. Her valuable assistance and effort have been indispensable in the completion of this book. The endless cooperation of the publisher, Williams & Wilkins, particularly Mr. James L. Sangston, Senior Editor of the publisher, in the preparation of this book is greatly appreciated.

Byrn Mawr, Pa.   **Edward K. Chung, M.D.**

Contents

Abbreviations

AF—atrial fibrillation
APC—atrial premature contraction
AVC—aberrant ventricular conduction
BBBB—bilateral bundle branch block
BFB—bifascicular block
BTS—brady-tachyarrhythmia syndrome
CHF—congestive heart failure
DC Shock—direct current shock
IHSS—idiopathic hypertrophic subaortic stenosis
LAHB—left anterior hemiblock
LBBB—left bundle branch block
LPHB—left posterior hemiblock
MAT—multifocal atrial tachycardia
MI—myocardial infarction
MVPS—mitral valve prolapse syndrome
PAT—paroxysmal atrial tachycardia
RBBB—right bundle branch block
SB—sinus bradycardia
SSS—sick sinus syndrome
TFB—trifascicular block
VF—ventricular fibrillation
VPC—ventricular premature contraction
VT—ventricular tachycardia
WPW Syndrome—Wolff-Parkinson-White syndrome

chapter 1

Sick Sinus Syndrome and Bradytachyarrhythmia Syndrome

Case 1

This ECG tracing was obtained from a 67-year-old man who had experienced several episodes of dizziness and near-syncope. He was not taking any medication.

What is your ECG diagnosis?

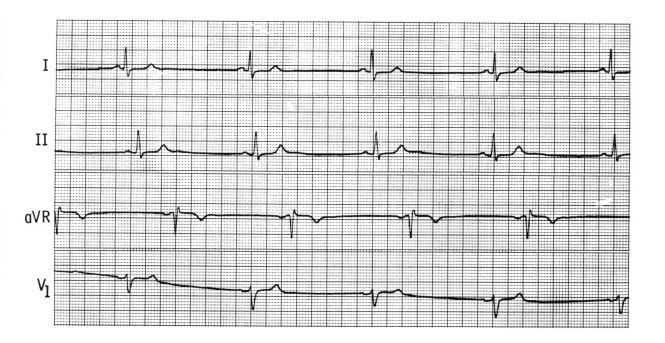

Case 1: Diagnosis

The cardiac rhythm is marked sinus bradycardia (SB) with a rate of 36 beats per minute. The diagnosis of sick sinus syndrome (SSS) should be always considered when dealing with unexplainable and persisting SB (rate slower than 40 beats per minute) not due to any drug. Ambulatory (Holter monitor) ECG to record the electrical activity of the heart for 24 hours without interruption is often indicated to confirm the diagnosis of SSS because the cardiac rhythm disorder may be transient and intermittent, so that the diagnostic ECG abnormalities may not be detected on a 12-lead ECG tracing (see Cases 2,3, and 9–12). When the clinical picture is equivocal and the electrocardiographic findings including the Holter monitor ECG result are not conclusive for the diagnosis of SSS, the electrophysiologic study is indicated. When the sinus node recovery time determined by the atrial pacing technique is found to be more than 1500 milliseconds, the diagnosis of SSS is certain (see Case 17).

Various ECG manifestations of SSS are summarized as follows:

1. Marked and persisting SB
2. Sinus arrest and/or sino-atrial (S-A) block
3. Drug (e.g., atropine, isoproterenol) resistant sinus bradyarrhythmias
4. Long pause following an atrial premature contraction (APC)
5. Prolonged sinus node recovery time (more than 1500 milliseconds) determined by atrial pacing
6. Chronic atrial fibrillation or repetitive occurrence of atrial fibrillation (less commonly atrial flutter):
    (a) with slow ventricular rate
    (b) preceded or followed by SB, sinus arrest, or S-A block
7. A-V junctional escape rhythm (with or without slow and unstable sinus activity)
8. Carotid sinus syncope (not every case)
9. Failure of restoration of sinus rhythm following cardioversion
10. Bradytachyarrhythmia syndrome (not every case)
11. Common coexisting A-V block and/or intraventricular block
12. Any combination of the above

Case 2

These Holter monitor rhythm strips were recorded from a 69-year-old woman with palpitations associated with dizziness. Her 12-lead ECG showed occasional ventricular premature contractions (VPCs), but was within normal limits otherwise (not shown here). She was not taking any drugs when the Holter monitor ECG was recorded.

1. *What is the cardiac rhythm diagnosis?*
2. *What is the treatment of choice?*

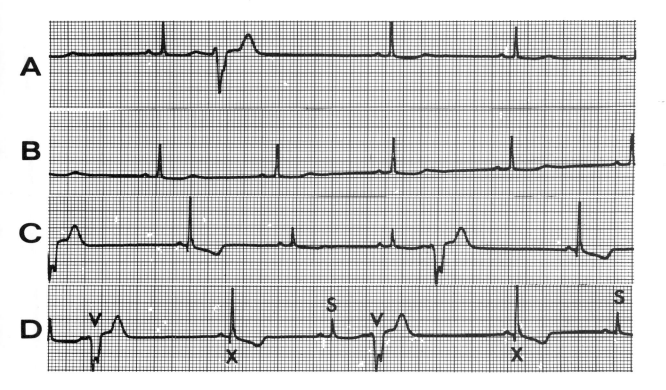

Case 2: Diagnosis

The cardiac rhythm strips A through D are not continuous. The cardiac rhythm is marked sinus bradycardia (rate: 43–55 beats per minute) with frequent VPCs (V) followed by ventricular escape beats (X). Note the sinus beats (S). Therefore, this Holter monitor ECG finding represents a bradytachyarrhythmia syndrome (BTS) secondary to SSS. In this ECG tracing, the expected A-V junctional escape beats failed to appear. Instead, a ventricular escape beat (X) appears following a long postectopic pause. This ECG finding most likely represents a diseased A-V node in addition to the sinus node dysfunction, a common occurrence.

The treatment of choice in this case is a permanent artificial pacemaker. If the VPCs are not suppressed by the artificial pacemaker, one or more antiarrhythmic drugs (e.g., quinidine, procainamide, etc.) may be required.

The therapeutic approach to SSS is summarized as follows:

Drug therapy alone for SSS is unsuccessful because:

(a) The agent for treatment of the tachyarrhythmia component is harmful for or aggravates the bradyarrhythmia component, and vice versa;

(b) There is a lack of long-term therapeutic effects of pharmacologic agents (e.g., atropine sulfate or isoproterenol) for bradyarrhythmias;

(c) There may be significant and intolerable side effects of all pharmacologic agents in many instances.

Currently, it is generally agreed that artificial pacemaker therapy is indicated in every significantly *symptomatic* patient in whom the symptoms are judged to be due to SSS. In addition, artificial pacing is to be considered in patients with far advanced SSS documented by ECG and/or electrophysiologic study, even if there is no significant symptom. It should be stressed, however, that it is necessary that the diagnosis of SSS be certain and that the arrhythmias are not due to unnecessary drugs being given to the patient.

1. *Artificial Pacemaker Therapy*

The ideal therapy is programmable pacing in which the most suitable pacing rate can be arranged according to the individual patient's need. Programmable pacing is ideal when there is a tachyarrhythmia component in SSS, so that pacing with a suitable rate may be capable of suppressing the tachyarrhythmia. Thus, the programmable pacing has been gradually replacing the conventional ventricular pacing mode in many medical centers in this country. On the other hand, a conventional demand ventricular pacemaker is still frequently used because the result is satisfactory in many cases with SSS.

The majority of individuals with this syndrome are elderly and the atrial contribution (kick) to increase the cardiac output is *not* essential for their daily activities. Therefore, ventricular pacing is sufficient to treat SSS in many elderly people. When the atrial kick is considered to be definitely needed for certain patients and when there is significant coexisting A-V conduction disturbance, and A-V sequential (bifocal) demand pacemaker is required.

When the coexisting A-V block is reasonably excluded, atrial pacing may be considered. One of the important advantages of atrial pacing (rate: 80–120 beats per minute) is that the atrial tachyarrhythmia component in BTS can be suppressed (up to 50% of cases) by pacing without the use of an antiarrhythmic agent. For this purpose, coronary sinus pacing is the preferred atrial pacemaker therapy. One of the disadvantageous aspects of coronary sinus pacing is that a suitable and constant pacing is not always predictable.

2. Digitalis and Antiarrhythmic Drug Therapy

As indicated earlier, antiarrhythmic drug therapy alone is unsatisfactory and often hazardous for SSS. However, antiarrhythmic drug therapy can be instituted with relative safety following implantation of a permanent pacemaker. Antiarrhythmic agents are often required for SSS because the tachyarrhythmia component is usually not suppressed by pacing alone, although atrial pacing may be capable of eliminating atrial tachyarrhythmias.

Indications for specific antiarrhythmic agents are similar to the general recommendations for various tachyarrhythmias which are not associated with SSS. Digitalis is the drug of choice for atrial fibrillation, flutter, or tachycardia with rapid ventricular response. Digitalis and diuretics may improve myocardial function and indirectly suppress the atrial tachyarrhythmias in patients with SSS associated with congestive heart failure. At times, propranolol may be added when atrial tachyarrhythmias with rapid ventricular response are not well controlled by digitalis alone. Quinidine is useful for the prevention of atrial tachyarrhythmias. When ventricular tachyarrhythmia is not controlled by artificial pacing, various drugs such as procainamide, quinidine, disopyramide, phenytoin, or propranolol may be tried as a single agent or combined.

Case 3

These Holter monitor ECG rhythm strips were obtained from a 59-year-old woman complaining of episodic dizziness. Cardiac examination, including a 12-lead ECG, was unremarkable (not shown here). She was not taking any medication.

1. *What is the cardiac rhythm diagnosis?*
2. *What is the treatment of choice?*

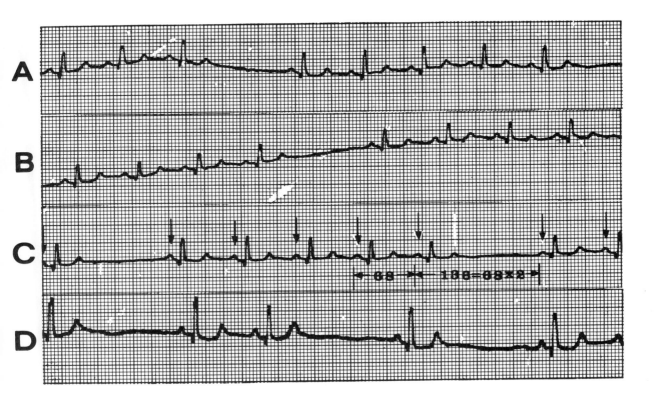

Case 3: Diagnosis

The cardiac rhythm strips A through D are not continuous. Note the sinus P waves (arrows). The cardiac rhythm is sinus arrhythmia with an intermittent Mobitz type II S-A block. Note that the long P-P interval is twice the basic P-P cycle (each number is 1/100 of a second). When a 2:1 S-A block occurs consecutively, as seen in strip D, the ventricular rate becomes extremely slow (36–38 beats per minute). Consequently, insufficient cardiac output can cause dizziness and even episodes of syncope.

As described earlier, S-A block is an expression of SSS (see Case 1). The treatment of choice is, of course, implantation of an artificial pacemaker.

Case 4

This ECG tracing was taken on an 80-year-old man who had fainted on several occasions. He was not taking any medication. Because of a very slow heart rate, the diagnosis of SSS is suspected.

1. *What is the ECG diagnosis?*
2. *What is the usual diagnostic approach to SSS?*

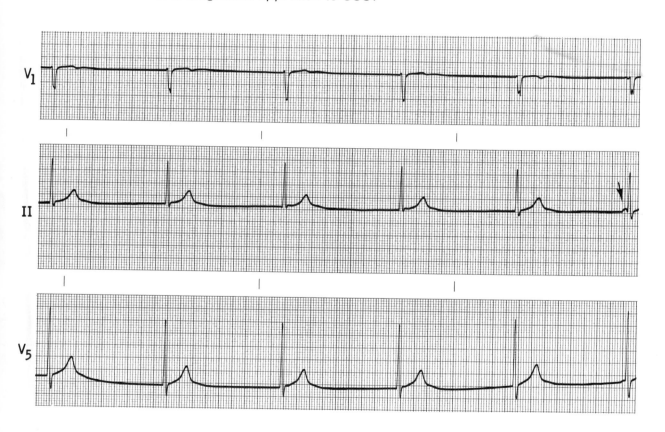

Case 4: Diagnosis

There is no discernible P wave in the entire ECG tracing except for one sinus P wave (indicated by arrow) which is not conducted to the ventricle. Thus, the cardiac rhythm diagnosis is A-V junctional escape rhythm with a rate of 34 beats per minute as a result of sinus arrest. The A-V junctional escape rhythm is slower than usual in this ECG tracing because of the diseased A-V node in addition to the diseased sinus node (common occurrence). Obviously, these ECG findings are manifestations of advanced SSS.

The diagnostic approach to SSS is summarized as follows:

Mild cases of SSS are not always easy to diagnose with certainty. A high index of suspicion is often necessary in many cases to reach a correct diagnosis during the early stage of SSS. Marked and persisting sinus bradycardia (*not* due to drugs) should always raise the possibility of SSS even in totally asymptomatic young individuals, including athletes.

1. *Clinical Manifestations*

The diagnosis of SSS cannot be made with certainty from clinical findings alone. However, SSS must be included among differential diagnoses when dealing with any patient with a history of syncope or near-syncope. Similarly, SSS should be suspected as a possible underlying disorder in any individual with unexplainable pulmonary edema, palpitations, or angina, particularly when these findings (singly or together) are associated with slow heart rate *not* due to drugs (e.g., digitalis, propranolol, etc.).

2. *Routine 12-lead ECG*

Diagnosis of advanced SSS can be confirmed by typical findings on a routine 12-lead ECG or long rhythm strips.

3. *Ambulatory (Holter Monitor) ECG*

When typical ECG findings of SSS are not documented on the routine 12-lead ECG because the finding is intermittent, the Holter monitor ECG is the best diagnostic tool.

4. *Carotid Sinus Stimulation (CSS) and Valsalva Maneuver*

Sinus arrest lasting more than 3 seconds with CSS is strongly suggestive of inappropriate sinus node responsiveness—SSS. As with CSS, the response to the Valsalva maneuver may be useful to demonstrate the sinus node dysfunction. That is, the Valsalva maneuver produces the expected changes in aortic pulse pressure, but causes little or no change in pulse rate. In contrast, the physiologic bradycardia of the elderly demonstrates the expected acceleration of the heart rate during the strain phase (phase III) and the subsequent slowing of the heart rate during the blood pressure overshoot (phase IV). However, it should be noted that these procedures provide no direct diagnostic evidence of the sinus node disease, but do give a clue to the functional status of the sinus node. Further investigation is often indicated in many cases.

5. *Cardioversion*

Needless to say, cardioversion is *not* a diagnostic method for SSS. However, a failure of restoration of sinus rhythm following termination of any ectopic tachyarrhythmia by the procedure is strongly diagnostic of SSS.

6. *Exercise ECG Test*

When the sinus rate does not increase significantly with the standard exercise ECG (e.g., treadmill), protocol SSS may be suspected providing that inappropriate sinus rate change is *not* influenced by drugs (e.g., propranolol). Healthy individuals in good physical condition (e.g., daily runners, athletes, etc.) may not show significant increment of heart rate with the exercise ECG protocol simply because of insufficient exercise load rather than the sinus node dysfunction.

7. *Drugs*

SSS is often suspected when any individual, particularly an elderly person, develops marked SB following administration of a small amount of digitalis or a beta-adrenergic blocking agent such as propranolol. SSS may be unmasked by these drugs. However, such a finding is not always reliable in diagnosis of SSS. Recently, atropine has been used to evaluate the response of the sinus node. Physiologic SB responds to the intravenous administration of atropine by a normal or exaggerated acceleration of the sinus rate. On the other hand, no significant increment of the sinus rate is observed in SSS following atropine administration. It has been suggested that when intravenous atropine sulfate (1–2 mg.) fails to increase the sinus rate beyond 90 beats per minute in SB, and when the sinus node recovery time remains prolonged by rapid (pacing rate: 120–140 beats per minute for 2–4 minutes) atrial pacing after atropine injection, diagnosis of SSS can be made. Similarly, diagnosis of SSS may be entertained when the sinus rate does not increase beyond 90-100 beats per minute in SB following intravenous administration of isoproterenol (1–2 μg./minute).

8. *Electrophysiologic Studies*

(See Case 17)

Case 5

This ECG tracing was obtained from a 76-year-old man with mild hypertension. He was not taking any drug.

1. *What is the cardiac rhythm diagnosis?*
2. *What is the treatment of choice?*

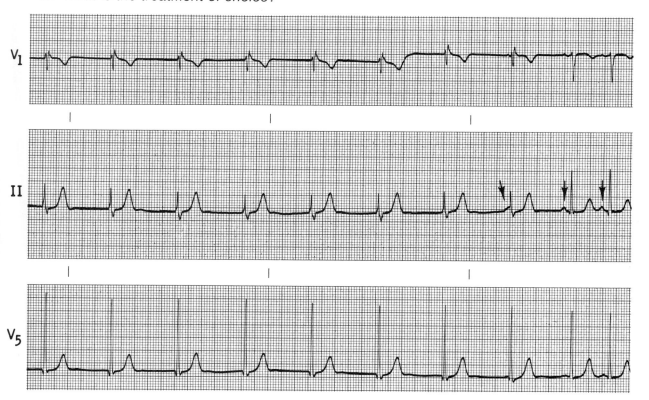

Case 5: Diagnosis

Arrows indicate P waves of sinus origin. The cardiac rhythm diagnosis is sinus arrhythmia (indicated by arrows) with sinus arrest leading to nonparoxysmal ventricular tachycardia (accelerated idioventricular rhythm or idioventricular tachycardia) with a rate of 60 beats per minute. The ectopic focus producing the tachycardia is most likely situated in one of the fascicles of the left bundle branch block (LBBB) system judging from the configuration of the QRS complex—a relatively narrow QRS complex showing incomplete right bundle branch block (RBBB) pattern. Thus, the precise diagnosis of the tachycardia is a "fascicular tachycardia." In a broad term, the fascicular tachycardia is a form of ventricular tachycardia. Note two normally conducted sinus beats (the last 2 beats).

No particular treatment is indicated for nonparoxysmal ventricular tachycardia or fascicular tachycardia, but the occurrence of a long sinus arrest is a serious clinical problem—a manifestation of SSS. Thus, the treatment of choice will be permanent pacemaker implantation (see Case 2). During careful history taking, this patient admitted that he had experienced frequent episodes of dizzy spells and occasional near-syncopes.

Case 6

This ECG tracing was taken on a 73-year-old woman with a permanent artificial pacemaker.

1. *What is your ECG diagnosis?*
2. *What was the underlying problem which required a permanent artificial pacemaker?*
3. *Is her artificial pacemaker working normally?*

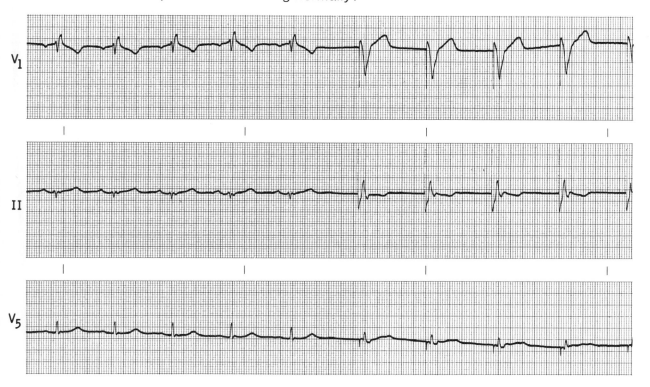

Case 6: Diagnosis

The cardiac rhythm is sinus (rate: 63 beats per minute) with first degree A-V block (P-R interval: 0.24 second) and intermittent demand ventricular pacemaker rhythm (rate: 54 beats per minute). The demand pacemaker takes over the ventricular activity when the sinus node fails to produce any cardiac impulse as a result of sinus arrest. Obviously, she required the artificial pacemaker for the treatment of SSS (see Case 2).

In addition, it is obvious to recognize RBBB. Common occurrence of various A-V conduction disturbances and/or intraventricular blocks in patients with SSS is a well-known fact.

The pacing rate is slower than usual in this patient because of a malfunctioning pulse generator which was implanted 6 years previously. The preset pacing rate was found to be 72 beats per minute. The malfunctioning pulse generator was replaced with a new unit.

Case 7

This ECG tracing was obtained from a 47-year-old man who fainted suddenly in the kitchen without any apparent reason. During careful history taking, he admitted that he had experienced frequent dizzy spells with occasional near-syncopal episodes associated with slow and irregular pulse. He was not taking any medication and otherwise had been apparently healthy. SSS was suspected clinically.

1. *What is your ECG diagnosis?*
2. *What are the usual clinical manifestations of SSS?*

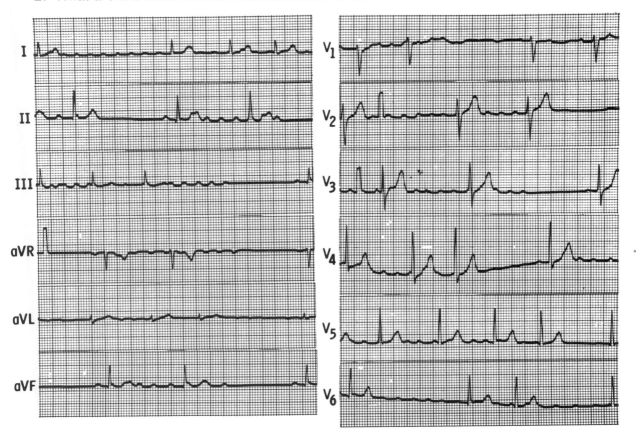

Case 7: Diagnosis

The cardiac rhythm is very unstable and slow sinus arrhythmia with SB and intermittent atrial flutter with advanced A-V block. Extremely slow ventricular rate during atrial flutter signifies advanced A-V block. Unquestionably, these ECG abnormalities are manifestations of advanced SSS. Permanent artificial pacemaker implantation was carried out without delay, and no further episode of near-syncope or syncope was observed.

The clinical manifestations in patients with SSS was fundamentally due to hypoperfusion of the vital organs, particularly the brain, heart, and kidney, as a result of the markedly slow ventricular rate which may or may not be associated with episodes of tachyarrhythmias.

There is no particular sexual preponderance in SSS, but the syndrome has been reported more frequently among elderly females than males. SSS may involve any age group, although it is primarily a disease of the elderly. The peak incidence of SSS has been reported to be in the 6th and 7th decades of life.

Clinical manifestations of SSS may be multifaceted, and they may occur only intermittently. The most common manifestations of advanced SSS are lightheadedness, near-syncope, or actual syncope, but in many mild cases, the patient may be totally asymptomatic or the syndrome may be difficult to recognize or evaluate in the early stage.

1. Cerebral Manifestations

In mild cases or in the early stage of SSS, diminished cerebral arterial blood flow may be manifested by generalized fatigue, muscle ache, or slight personality changes including irritability, intermittent memory loss, and insomnia. When SSS has further progressed, cerebral manifestations may include slurred speech, paresis, erroneous judgment, lightheadedness, and near-syncope followed by fainting. Severe cerebral manifestations such as syncope or near-syncope are almost always due to marked slowing of the heart rate or cardiac arrest; the tachycardia component seldom produces significant cerebral symptoms.

Since SSS is primarily a disease of the elderly, the cerebral manifestations are frequently misinterpreted as cerebrovascular accidents or simply as "senility." Syncope or near-syncope has been reported to occur in 40–70% of the patients with SSS. The incidence of dizziness was reported to be 6–7% of the cases with SSS.

2. Cardiac Manifestations

Various cardiac manifestations are the second most common finding in SSS. In the early stage of mild SSS, cardiac manifestations other than a slow heart rate or mixture of slow and rapid cardiac rhythms may be completely absent. The three most common cardiac manifestations in SSS include palpitations, increased signs of congestive heart failure (CHF), and increased angina. In some instances, a sudden occurrence of or episodic acute pulmonary edema may be the first sign of SSS, because the patient may not seek medical attention during the mild stage. Feelings of palpitations may be due to the extremely slow rhythm itself (e.g., sinus bradycardia or atrial fibrillation with advanced A-V block), irregular rhythm, or a mixture of slow and rapid rhythms (bradytachyarrhythmia syndrome). Most patients experience palpitations when the cardiac rhythm suddenly changes—from slow to rapid or vice versa. The occurrence of the three common cardiac manifestations (palpitations, angina, and CHF) of SSS are interrelated, and one symptom frequently aggravates the others.

In far advanced cases of SSS, the patients may develop prolonged cardiac arrest or ventricular fibrillation leading to death.

3. Other Manifestations

Various nonspecific manifestations such as oliguria, gastrointestinal distress, etc., are not uncommon in SSS, but these findings are usually secondary to hypoperfusion of the heart itself.

A 64-year-old woman was evaluated at the cardiac clinic because of very slow heart rate associated with mild CHF. She was not taking any medication.

1. *What is your ECG diagnosis?*
2. *What is the treatment of choice?*

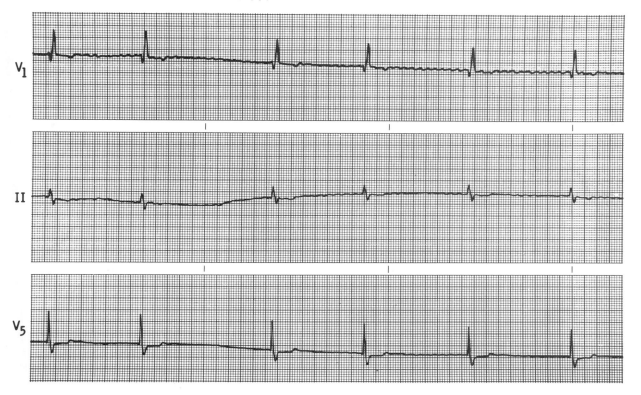

Case 8: Diagnosis

The cardiac rhythm is atrial fibrillation with very slow ventricular response (ventricular rate: 30–35 beats per minute) due to advanced A-V block. Note that some R-R intervals are regular because of intermittent A-V junctional escape rhythm. These ECG abnormalities indicate far advanced SSS (see Case 1). The diagnosis of SSS is almost certain when any individual develops atrial fibrillation with slow ventricular rate (slower than 60 beats per minute) without any medication (e.g., digitalis or propranolol). In SSS, atrial fibrillation with advanced A-V block is frequently preceded by marked SB with or without first degree A-V block, and intermittent sinus arrest or S-A block (see Case 1).

In addition, there is RBBB in this ECG tracing. It has been well documented that SSS is often associated with various intraventricular conduction disturbances including hemiblocks, RBBB, LBBB, and bifascicular or trifascicular block because the same underlying disease process (usually degenerative sclerotic change) involves the sinus node as well as bundle branch system—Purkinje fibers. The rate of A-V junctional escape rhythm is markedly slow in SSS because the sinus node as well as the A-V node dysfunctions altogether.

The treatment of choice is permanent artificial pacemaker implantation on this patient. When CHF is found to be a manifestation of SSS, acceleration of the heart rate by artificial pacing is sufficient to treat the heart failure in most cases without using diuretics or digitalis (see Case 2).

These Holter monitor ECG rhythm strips were obtained from a 62-year-old woman with frequent episodes of dizziness. She had almost fainted on several occasions. She was found to have mild hypertension, but she was not taking any drugs when the Holter monitor ECG was recorded. Her 12-lead ECG revealed a sinus bradycardia with sinus arrhythmia (rate: 48–57 beats per minute) and occasional VPCs with left ventricular hypertrophy (not shown here).

1. *What is the cardiac rhythm diagnosis?*
2. *What is the treatment of choice?*

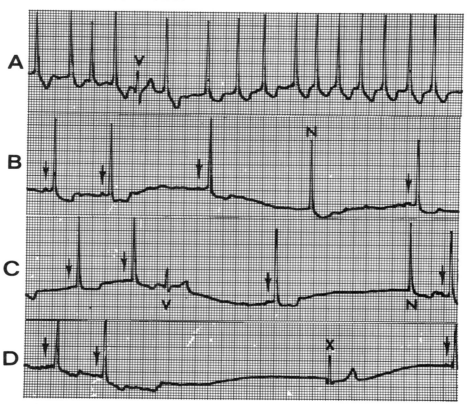

Case 9: Diagnosis

Strips A through D are not continuous. Note the sinus P waves (arrows). The cardiac rhythm is markedly unstable sinus mechanism, with periods of extreme sinus bradycardia and sinus arrest, leading to occasional A-V junctional escape beats (N) as well as ventricular escape beats (X). In addition, paroxysmal atrial fibrillation is recorded (strip A), and there are occasional VPCs (V).

The cardiac rhythm diagnosis is a good example of a bradytachyarrhythmia syndrome (BTS) secondary to a far advanced SSS. The treatment of choice is, of course, a permanent pacemaker implantation.

Case 10

A 77-year-old man was referred to a cardiologist for the evaluation of many syncope episodes. He was not taking any drugs.

1. *What is the 12-lead ECG diagnosis?*
2. *What is the Holter monitor ECG diagnosis?*
3. *What is the treatment of choice?*

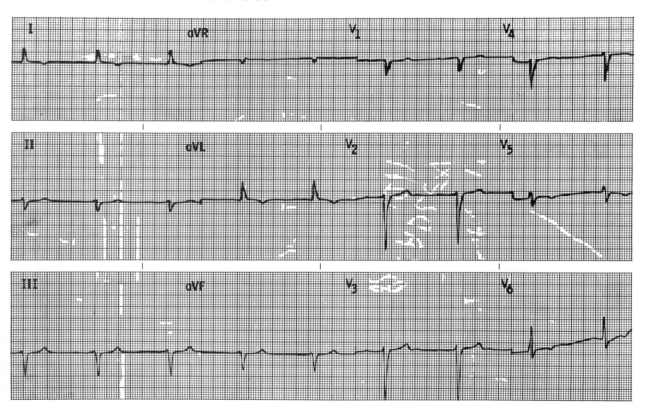

Case 10: Diagnosis

12-lead ECG: The 12-lead ECG reveals sinus bradycardia (SB) (rate: 48 beats minute), with a first degree A-V block (the P-R interval: 0.32 second) and a left anterior hemiblock (QRS axis: − 50 degrees) with a nonspecific abnormality of the T waves. Obviously, the above ECG finding does not explain his symptom, syncope episodes. Therefore, the Holter monitor ECG was obtained.

Holter Monitor ECG: The strips A through E are not continuous. The basic rhythm is again SB, with a first degree A-V block. Frequent multifocal ventricular premature contractions (VPCs) with intermittent ventricular tachycardia are easily recognized. Needless to say, these ECG findings are typical example of a serious BTS due to an advanced SSS. Implantation of a permanent artificial pacemaker is, of course, the treatment of choice. One or more (usually quinidine or procainamide) antiarrhythmic drugs may be needed if the tachyarrhythmia component persists after pacing.

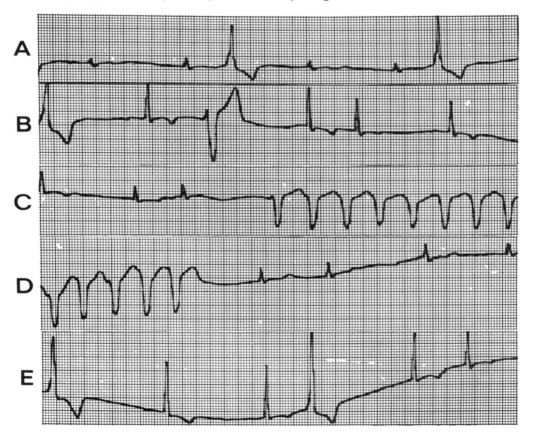

Case 11

A 73-year-old man was seen in the cardiologist's office for evaluation of dizziness. The physical examination showed a normal elderly male without demonstrable heart disease or cerebrovascular disorder. His 12-lead ECG was definitely abnormal, but the finding was not sufficient to explain his dizziness. Therefore, the Holter monitor ECG was obtained. He was not taking any drugs.

1. *What is the 12-lead ECG diagnosis?*
2. *What is the cardiac rhythm diagnosis on the Holter monitor ECG?*
3. *What is the treatment of choice?*

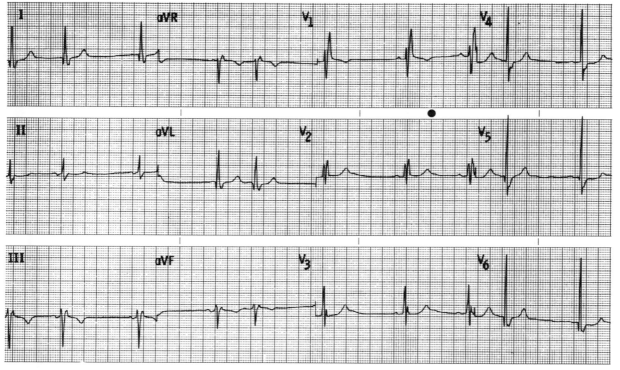

J.S., 73 M. (#1) - DIZZINESS

Case 11: Diagnosis

12-lead ECG: The underlying cardiac rhythm is SB (rate: 50 beats per minute), with occasional atrial premature contractions (APCs). The diagnosis of RBBB is obvious on the basis of an RR' pattern of the QRS complexes in leads V_1 and V_2, with slurred and deep S waves in leads I, aVL, and V_{4-6}. In addition, left ventricular hypertrophy is suggested by voltage criteria.

Holter Monitor ECG: Strips A through C are not continuous. The P waves are not clearly discernible (a not uncommon finding in elderly individuals), but from the finding on the 12-lead ECG, the cardiac rhythm is most likely sinus. There are frequent APCs, with atrial group beats and paroxysmal atrial tachycardia (PAT). Note also the occasional ventricular escape beats (X). In addition, it is interesting that a very long pause follows the termination of PAT (strip A). This finding is a reliable sign of an abnormally prolonged sinus node recovery time. Thus, a diagnosis of SSS can be made. The occurrence of ventricular escape beats (X) following a pause is indirect evidence of a diseased A-V node because the expected A-V junctional escape beats fail to appear. It is well known that SSS is often associated with a diseased A-V node, since the same process often involves the sinus node as well as the A-V node.

  The Holter monitor ECG findings on this patient show BTS, which is a manifestation of advanced SSS (see Case 1). The treatment of choice is implantation of a permanent pacemaker. When atrial tachycardia recurs following artificial pacing, one or more antiarrhythmic drugs (e.g., propranolol, quinidine, digitalis) may be indicated (see Case 2).

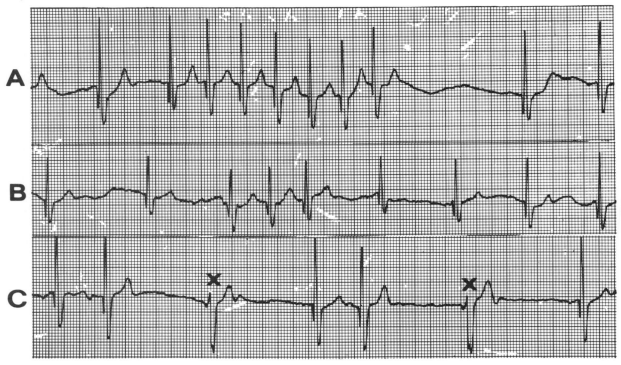

J.S., 73 M. (#2) – Dizziness

Case 12

A 73-year-old woman was referred to a cardiologist because of palpitations and dizziness. She was not taking any drugs when the Holter monitor ECG was ordered. The 12-lead ECG showed an atrial fibrillation (AF) with a relatively slow ventricular rate of 55–65 beats per minute and occasional VPCs (not shown here).

1. *What is the cardiac rhythm diagnosis?*
2. *What is the treatment of choice?*

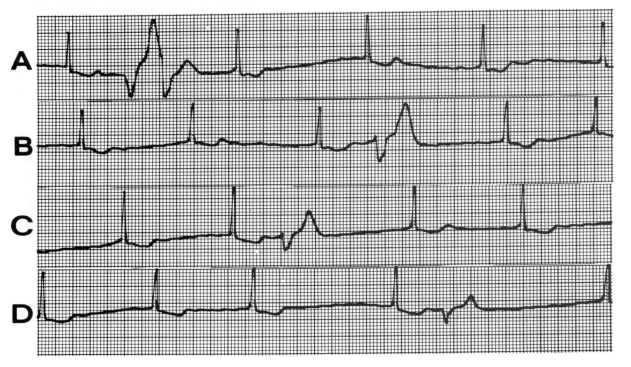

Case 12: Diagnosis

Strips A through D are not continuous. The cardiac rhythm is AF with an advanced A-V block producing a slow ventricular rate (42–46 beats per minute) and frequent VPCs, with ventricular group beats. Note that the ventricular cycle is *not* regular, and, therefore, the diagnosis of complete A-V block *cannot* be made. Under this circumstance the term "advanced" or "high-degree" A-V block is used to express the slow but irregular ventricular cycle in AF.

This ECG finding is another expression of a BTS due to an advanced SSS. It should be noted that chronic AF with advanced A-V block is a common manifestation of advanced SSS (see Case 1).

A permanent artificial pacemaker was implanted, with excellent results in this patient.

Case 13

A 64-year-old man was brought to the cardiac clinic for the evaluation of his frequent dizzy spells associated with occasional near-syncope. He was not taking any drug. He stated that his symptoms occur more commonly when he turns the neck or shaves with an electric shaver. These ECG rhythm strips were obtained during and after carotid sinus stimulation. Leads II-a, b, and c are continuous.

1. *What is your diagnosis?*
2. *What is the treatment of choice?*

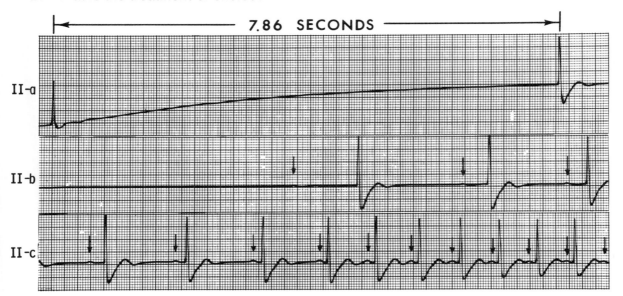

Case 13: Diagnosis

The basic rhythm is sinus (indicated by arrows), but a long sinus arrest with ventricular standstill (7.86 seconds) is produced by carotid sinus stimulation (CSS). This is a good example of hypertensive reaction to CSS. This phenomenon is termed "carotid sinus syncope," which is often a manifestation of SSS (see Case 1). Note occasional A-V junctional escape beats during a long sinus arrest until sinus rhythm progressively speeds up its rate. The P-R intervals also progressively shorten until a normal P-R interval is established.

The treatment of choice is, of course, permanent pacemaker implantation (see Case 2). It should be noted that artificial pacemaker implantation is the treatment of choice for all patients with carotid sinus syncope.

Case 14

These ECG rhythm strips were obtained from a 30-year-old woman with dizzy spells and near-syncopes. Surgical correction of atrial septal defect (ostium secundum type) was carried out 10 years previously, and the postoperative recovery was uneventful until several weeks previous, when she began to experience the above-mentioned symptoms. She was not taking any drug.

   1. *What is your ECG diagnosis?*
   2. *What is the treatment of choice?*

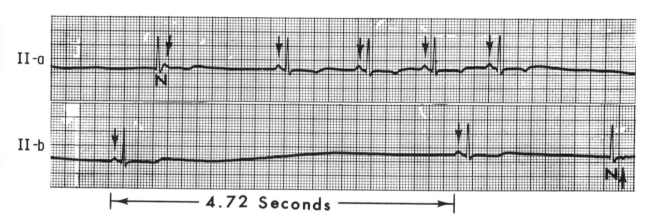

Case 14: Diagnosis

Leads II-a and b are continuous. Downward arrows indicate sinus P waves. The cardiac rhythm is sinus arrhythmia with a long sinus arrest (4.72 seconds) and occasional A-V junctional escape beats (marked N). Note a retrograde P wave (indicated by upward arrow). These ECG findings represent advanced SSS (see Case 1). It has been shown that some patients with atrial septal defect (either ostium secundum or primum type) progressively develop dysfunction of sinus node over 10–15 years postoperatively, leading to SSS.

The treatment of choice is, needless to say, permanent artificial pacemaker implantation (shown in this page). The ECG tracing shown in this page reveals a demand ventricular pacemaker rhythm with a rate of 72 beats per minute.

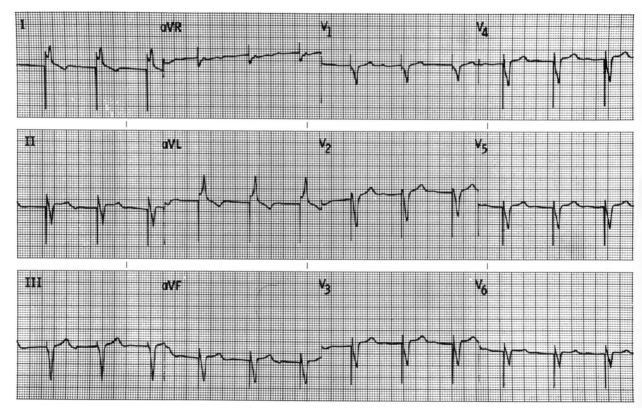

Case 15

This ECG tracing was obtained from a 79-year-old man with frequent episodes of near-syncope. He was not taking any drug. Leads II-a and b and leads V₁-a and b are continuous in each given lead.

1. *What is your ECG diagnosis?*
2. *What is the treatment of choice?*

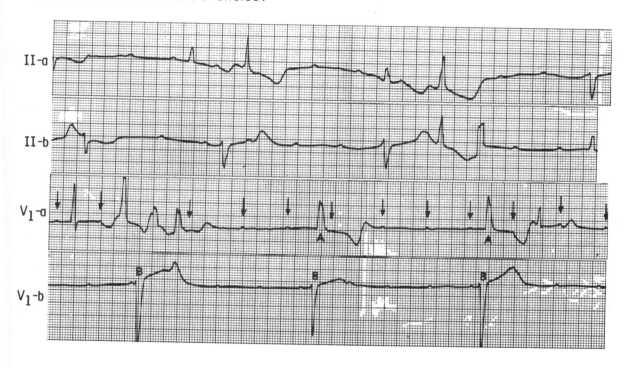

Case 15: Diagnosis

Arrows indicate sinus P waves. The cardiac rhythm is sinus (rate: 86 beats per minute), with complete A-V block producing extremely slow ventricular escape rhythms (rate: 22–25 beats per minute) arising from 2 foci (marked A and B). In addition, there are frequent multifocal VPCs with group beats. These ECG findings represent BTS. It should be noted, however, that these ECG findings are *not* a manifestation of SSS. In other words, the sinus node functions normally in this patient.

The site of A-V block in this patient is below the His bundle—infra-His block. Thus, complete A-V block in this patient represents complete bilateral bundle branch block (BBBB), meaning complete trifascicular block (TFB; see Chapters 2 and 3).

The treatment of choice is permanent pacemaker implantation for BTS. Slightly faster pacing rate (80–120 beats per minute) may be required in order to suppress the VPCs. One or more antiarrhythmic agents (e.g., quinidine, procainamide, propranolol, etc.) may be indicated after artificial pacing when VPCs persist.

Case 16

These rhythm strips were obtained from a 57-year-old man with acute anterior myocardial infarction. Leads II-a, b, and c are not continuous.

1. *What is the ECG diagnosis?*
2. *What is the treatment of choice?*

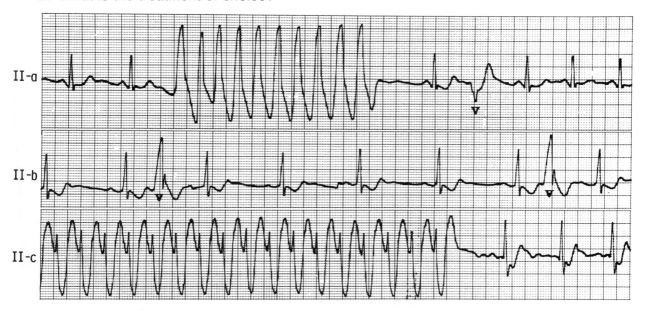

II-a

II-b

II-c

Case 16: Diagnosis

The basic rhythm indicates sinus arrhythmia with an area of sinus bradycardia (SB) (rate: 50–85 beats per minute). There are two types of QRS complex during tachycardias with different rates. Thus, paroxysmal bidirectional ventricular tachycardia is diagnosed. The ventricular rates in these tachycardias are 200 beats per minute (lead II-a) and 170 beats per minute (lead II-c). Note two types of VPC (marked V) during sinus rhythm (lead II-b).

Thus, the final ECG diagnosis is bradytachyarrhythmia syndrome (BTS). The initial treatment of choice for this patient is intravenous injection of Xylocaine (lidocaine), followed by intravenous infusion of the drug. If the drug therapy is found to be ineffective, however, artificial pacing with slight overdriving pacing rate (80–120 beats per minute) should be considered.

Case 17

A 45-year-old woman with amyloidosis developed marked slowing of the heart rate associated with CHF and dizziness. SSS was suspected by reviewing her ECG findings in conjunction with the clinical picture. Electrophysiologic study was performed.

1. *What is your ECG diagnosis?*
2. *What is the common electrophysiologic study to confirm the diagnosis of SSS?*

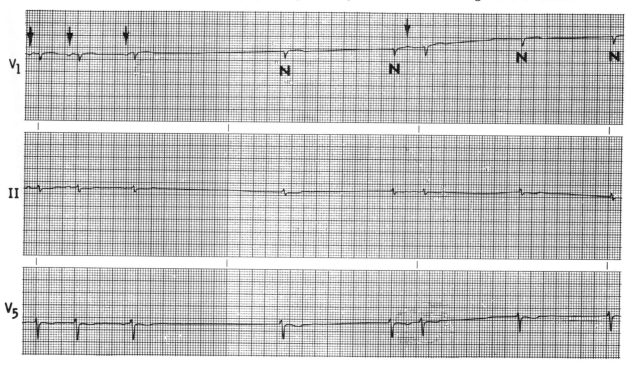

Case 17: Diagnosis

The ECG tracing shows a long period (4.44 seconds) of spontaneous sinus arrest and unstable A-V junctional escape rhythm (marked N). It is interesting to note that the first A-V junctional escape interval is also significantly prolonged. Arrows indicate P waves.

The tracing shown on this page reveals the sinus node recovery time by atrial pacing with a rate of 120 beats per minute. The sinus node recovery time is markedly prolonged (the interval from the upward arrow to the downward arrow—13.68 seconds) because of SSS. Note that the first A-V junctional escape interval (marked N) is also markedly prolonged because of coexisting A-V nodal dysfunction. Leads V_{1-a} and b and leads II-a and b are continuous in each given lead.

Electrophysiologic studies for the diagnosis of SSS are summarized as follows:

1. *Determination of Sinus Node Recovery Time by Atrial Pacing*

Among various electrophysiologic studies, determination of the sinus node recovery time (postpacing pause) by rapid atrial pacing is the most reliable provocative test for indirect evidence of SSS. It can be obtained by the use of a pervenous right atrial pacing catheter and the conventional electrocardiographic recordings. The artificial pacing can be performed by placing the pacing catheter either within the coronary sinus or at the junction of the superior vena cava and right atrium, whichever location provides the most effective and consecutive atrial capture. The initial pacing rate is usually 90 beats per minute, and it is progressively increased thereafter by 10 beats every 2–4 minutes up to 150 beats per minute. The pacing is terminated suddenly at the end of each period, and the postpacing pause (the interval from the last pacing spike to the onset of the next sinus P wave) is measured. When there is complete absence of sinus P waves (atrial standstill) following the termination of pacing, the first A-V junctional escape interval (the interval from the last pacing spike to the first A-V junctional escape beat) is measured. Atrial pacing must be restarted immediately, however, when there is complete cardiac arrest for 4 seconds in order to avoid a syncopal episode.

The postpacing pause is expected to occur in individuals with normal as well as diseased sinus nodes, and this electrophysiologic phenomenon is comparable to the post-tachyarrhythmia pause. The diseased sinus node, needless to say, requires abnormally long recovery time until the automaticity as a primary pacemaker is re-established. Thus, it has been documented that there is a clear distinction between normal and abnormal responses.

It has been reported that the actual sinus node recovery time following termination of atrial pacing is closely related to the resting sinus rate—the slower the resting sinus rate, the longer the maximum postpacing pause. When the resting sinus rate is between 75 and 85 beats per minute, the maximum normal postpacing pause is estimated to be 115 and 128% of the resting cycle length (postpacing pause: 800–900 milliseconds). In sinus bradycardia (rate: 45–60 beats per minute), the maximum normal postpacing pause is expected to be much longer, and abnormally prolonged sinus node suppression can be easily recognized. In sinus rhythm with a rate of 60 beats per minute (cycle length: 1000 milliseconds), the postpacing pause showing 125% or greater of the resting value (1250 milliseconds) is strongly suggestive of abnormal function of the sinus node. When the resting sinus rate is 45 beats per minute (cycle length: 1420 milliseconds), the postpacing pause of 1700 milliseconds or greater is diagnostic of abnormal function of the sinus node, although the percentage increase is only 120%. In severe SSS, the postpacing pause may reach between 2000 and 6000 milliseconds.

Narula et al. proposed use of the corrected sinus node recovery time (CSRT)—the difference between the postpacing pause and the resting sinus P-P cycle. Normal maximum CSRT is calculated to be 525 milliseconds or less, whereas the abnormal CSRT is calculated to be 1880 ± 1079 milliseconds.

It should be noted that although the determination of the sinus node recovery time by atrial pacing remains the best indirect diagnostic approach for SSS, the test may still be a false-negative in some instances. Also, the demonstration of an abnormally prolonged recovery time does not establish the diagnosis of SSS; SSS is established only when significant symptoms are due to abnormal sinus node function.

2. Determination of Sinoatrial Conduction Time by Atrial Extrastimulus Technique

By another method of electrophysiologic study, the sinoatrial conduction times (SACT) were measured indirectly by atrial extrastimulus technique. In one study, prolonged (more than 152 milliseconds) calculated SACT was associated with high incidence of sinus node and/or atrial disease. On the other hand, SACT was not significantly different between the control group and the patients with SSS studied by others.

3. His Bundle Electrocardiography

Since SSS is often associated with various abnormalities in the impulse formation and conduction elsewhere in the heart, His bundle electrocardiography can provide useful information. For example, abnormal electrophysiologic properties within the A-V junction may indirectly support the diagnosis of SSS. In addition, by recognizing the coexisting conduction disturbance, a specific type of artificial pacing may be selected for a given patient with SSS.

A permanent artificial pacemaker was implanted with a good result on this patient.

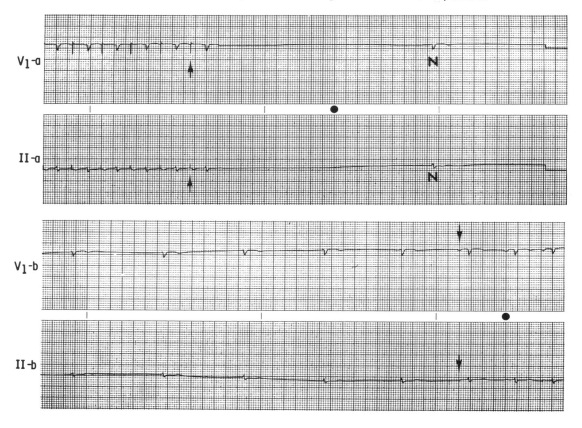

Case 18

This ECG tracing was obtained from a 74-year-old woman with dizziness associated with slow pulse rate. She was not taking any drug.

What is your ECG diagnosis?

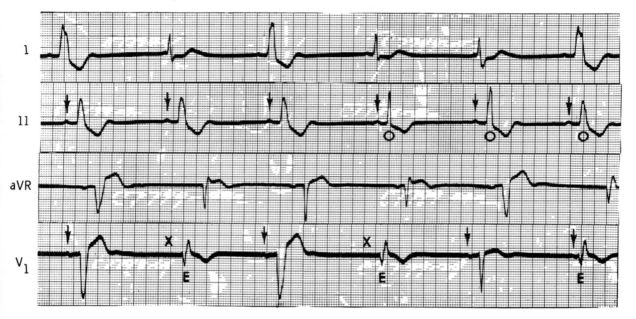

Case 18: Diagnosis

Arrows indicate sinus P waves. The cardiac rhythm is marked SB (rate: 35 beats per minute) with intermittent Mobitz type-II S-A block (marked X) and frequent ventricular escape beats (marked E). Note frequent ventricular fusion beats (marked 0). The evidence of left LBBB is obvious. These ECG findings indicate advanced SSS (see Case 1). Coexisting A-V nodal disease is strongly considered because the expected A-V junctional escape beats fail to appear during S-A block. Instead, ventricular escape beats (marked E) are observed in this patient. Common occurrence of various intraventricular blocks in SSS is well recognized.

chapter 2

Intraventricular Conduction Disturbance

Case 19

These ECG rhythm strips were taken on a 58-year-old man as a part of an annual check-up. He was not taking any drug and was found to be apparently healthy.

What is your ECG diagnosis?

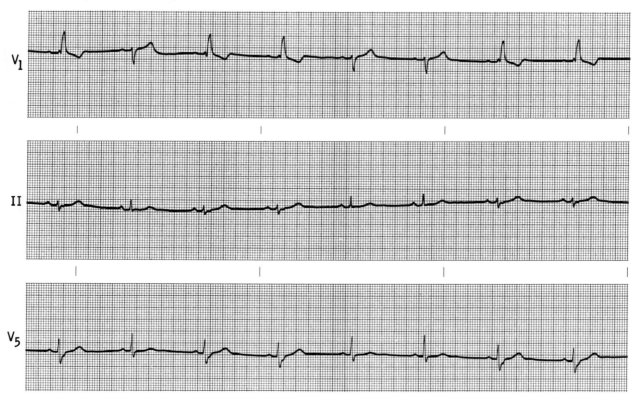

Case 19: Diagnosis

The cardiac rhythm is sinus bradycardia (SB) with a rate of 52 beats per minute. It is obvious that there are two kinds of QRS complexes. The ECG finding is due to intermittent right bundle branch block (RBBB). Superficially, frequent ventricular premature contractures (VPCs) with group beats are simulated. Needless to say, intermittent RBBB has no clinical significance, but it eventually leads to fixed RBBB. The occurrence of intermittent RBBB in this case does not seem to be related to the heart rate. Thus, intermittent RBBB is said to be rate-independent under this circumstance.

Case 20

This ECG tracing was recorded on a 71-year-old man with a previous history of extensive anterior myocardial infarction (MI) as well as diaphragmatic (inferior) myocardial infarction. He was not taking any drug other than hydrochlorothiazide 50 mg. every other day for mild heart failure. He had recovered from the heart attack almost completely.

1. *What is your ECG diagnosis?*
2. *What is the treatment of choice?*

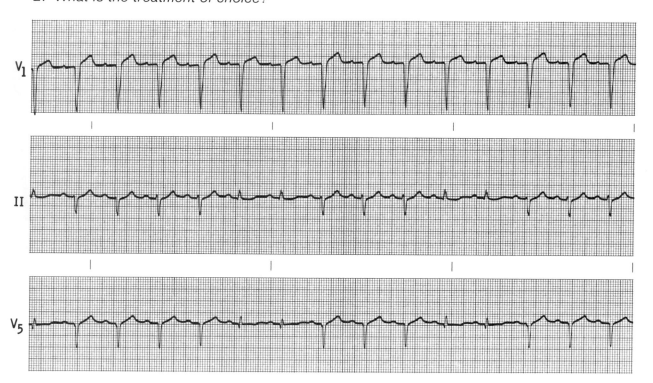

Case 20: Diagnosis

The cardiac rhythm is sinus rhythm (rate: 87 beats per minute) with slight first degree A-V block (P-R interval: 0.22 second). Note that there are two types of the QRS complexes as a result of intermittent shift of the QRS axis. Namely, this ECG finding indicates intermittent left anterior hemiblock (LAHB). The QRS axis during LAHB is estimated to be about −50 degrees. In addition, evidence of old anterior and diaphragmatic MI can be recognized (only 3 leads are shown).

The diagnostic criteria of LAHB are as follows:
(1) Marked left axis deviation (QRS axis −45 to −90°)
(2) Small q wave in lead I and small r wave in lead III
(3) Little or no prolongation of the QRS interval
(4) No evidence of other factors responsible for left axis deviation (true or pseudo)

The fundamental mechanism responsible for the production of marked left axis deviation in LAHB is diagrammatically illustrated on this page. When both anterior and posterior divisions of left bundle branch system are intact (diagram A), the left ventricle is activated via both divisions (vectors 1 and 2), so that the resultant forces of vectors 1 and 2 will produce vector 3. When one of two divisions of the left bundle branch system is blocked, however, the impulses must travel through the intact division only. That is, in anterior hemiblock (diagram B), vector 1 is no longer present, and as a result, the left ventricle is activated via intact posterior division (vector 2). In this case, the electrical axis shifts to the left and superiorly (marked left axis deviation). For the same reason, posterior hemiblock (diagram C) produces right axis deviation because the left ventricle is activated via intact anterior division (vector 1). KEY: RB, right bundle branch; AVN, A-V node; LAD, left anterior division; LPD, left posterior division.

As far as the clinical significance is concerned, LAHB alone has no significance. Accordingly, no treatment is indicated. Chronic LAHB is considered to be due to a sclerotic-degenerative process in the left anterior fascicle of the left bundle branch, as seen in any other portion of the Purkinje system. However, LAHB of acute onset is usually due to direct damage of the left anterior fascicle as a result of anteroseptal MI.

Superficially, intermittent LAHB resembles VPCs with group beats or even a short run of slow ventricular tachycardia (nonparoxysmal ventricular tachycardia, accelerated idioventricular rhythm, or idioventricular tachycardia; see Cases 86, 107, and 108).

Intermittent LAHB has no clinical significance, and accordingly, no treatment is necessary.

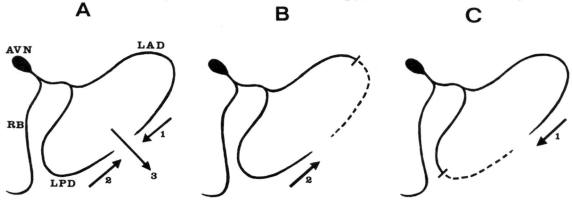

DIAGRAM: HEMIBLOCKS

Case 21

These ECG rhythm strips were obtained from a 30-year-old man with aortic stenosis.

What is your ECG diagnosis?

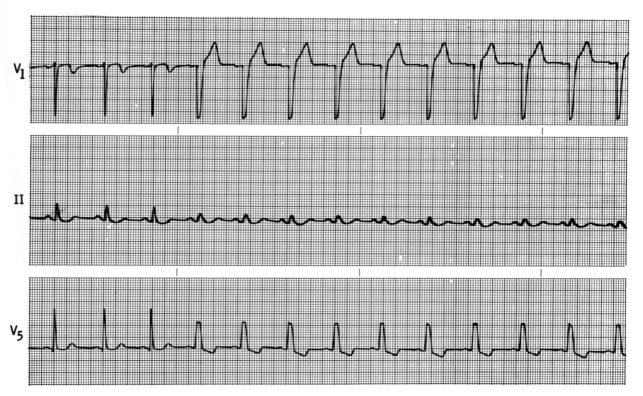

Case 21: Diagnosis

The cardiac rhythm is sinus rhythm with a rate of 80 beats per minute. There are two types of QRS complexes because of intermittent left bundle branch block (LBBB). The cardiac rhythm during LBBB closely mimics ectopic rhythm such as nonparoxysmal ventricular tachycardia (accelerated ventricular rhythm) or parasystolic ventricular tachycardia (see Cases 86, 107, and 108).

The term "rate-dependent" bundle branch block is used when right or left bundle block occurs during faster ventricular rate. Otherwise, intermittent bundle branch block is said to be "rate-independent," as seen in this case. In general, rate-dependent bundle branch block eventually becomes rate-independent bundle branch block, which finally leads to a fixed and chronic bundle branch block. LBBB is common in patients with aortic stenosis.

Case 22

This ECG tracing was obtained from a 65-year-old woman with essential hypertension. She had been taking hydrochlorothiazide 50 mg. once daily for several years.

What is your ECG diagnosis?

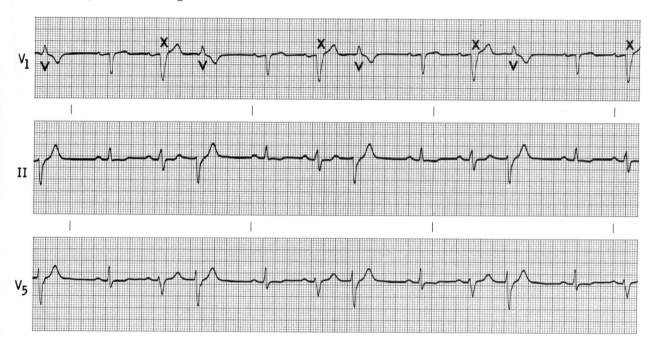

Case 22: Diagnosis

The cardiac rhythm is normal sinus rhythm with a rate of 72 beats per minute. It is obvious that there are 3 kinds of QRS complexes which occur on a regular basis. This ECG demonstrates frequent VPCs, causing ventricular trigeminy (marked V) and rate-dependent LBBB (marked X). The left bundle branch system recovers from its refractoriness following a postectopic pause leading to a normal conduction. In addition, left atrial enlargement is suggested. LBBB and left atrial enlargement are common in hypertensive patients.

Case 23

A 50-year-old obese woman was admitted to the coronary care unit because of severe chest pain associated with cold sweat of a few hours in duration. She gave a history of a heart attack about 1 year previously. The ECG tracing shown on this page (tracing A) was taken on admission, whereas another ECG tracing (tracing B), shown on the reverse side, was recorded several hours later.

1. *What is your diagnosis of both ECG tracings?*
2. *What is the underlying conduction abnormality found by reviewing both ECG tracings?*
3. *What is the treatment of choice?*

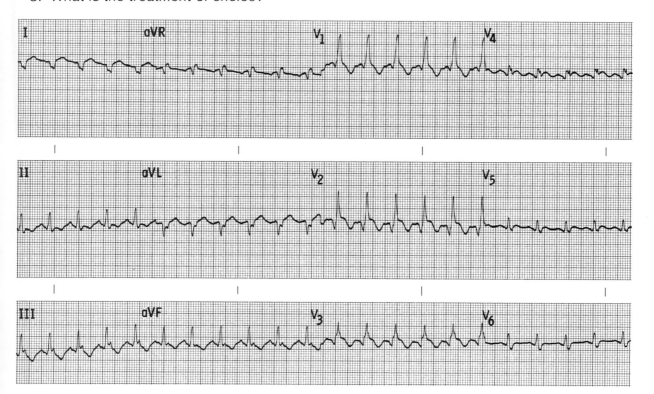

Case 23: Diagnosis

Tracing A: The cardiac rhythm is sinus tachycardia with a rate of 128 beats per minute. The ECG abnormalities include acute extensive anterior MI and bifascicular block (BFB) consisting of right bundle branch block (RBBB) and left posterior hemiblock (LPHB). In addition, old diaphragmatic MI is strongly suggested. BFB is, of course, a form of incomplete bilateral bundle branch block (BBBB). Note marked right axis deviation of the QRS complexes (axis: +120 degrees) as a result of LPHB (see Case 20).

Tracing B: This ECG tracing taken several hours later again shows sinus tachycardia with a rate of 132 beats per minute. It should be noted that the QRS axis is markedly shifted leftward (QRS axis: −90 degrees). This ECG finding represents left anterior hemiblock (LAHB). Thus, the ECG abnormalities in this tracing include acute extensive anterior MI associated with BFB consisting of RBBB and LAHB and probable diaphragmatic MI.

When both ECG tracings (A and B) are reviewed, it is obvious that the fundamental conduction abnormality is incomplete trifascicular block (TFB) which is incomplete BBBB.

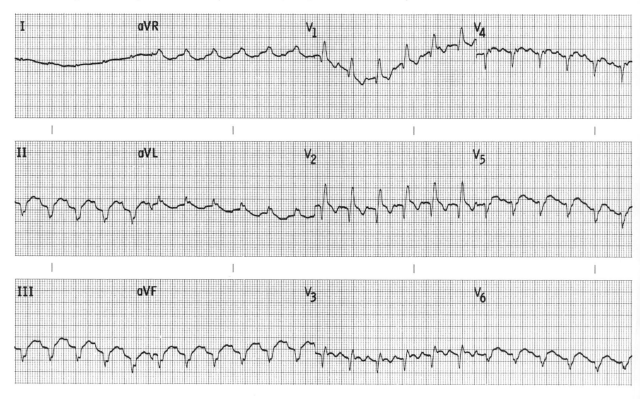

The diagnostic criteria of BBBB are summarized as follows:

Diagnostic Criteria of Bilateral Bundle Branch Block
(Bifascicular and Trifascicular Block)

(1) RBBB with LAHB
(2) RBBB with LPHB
(3) Alternating LBBB and RBBB
(4) LBBB or RBBB with first or second degree A-V block (in most cases)
(5) LBBB or RBBB with prolonged H-V interval (more than 70 milliseconds)
(6) LBBB on one occasion and RBBB on another occasion
(7) Mobitz type II A-V block
(8) Complete (infra-nodal) A-V block with ventricular escape rhythm
(9) Any combination of the above findings

The treatment of choice in this patient is immediate insertion of a prophylactic artificial pacemaker followed by permanent pacemaker implantation

Case 24

This ECG tracing was obtained from a 33-year-old obese woman who has been a heavy cigarette smoker for more than 10 years. She was admitted to the coronary care unit because a heart attack was suspected clinically. She was not taking any medication.

1. *What is your ECG diagnosis?*
2. *What is the treatment of choice?*

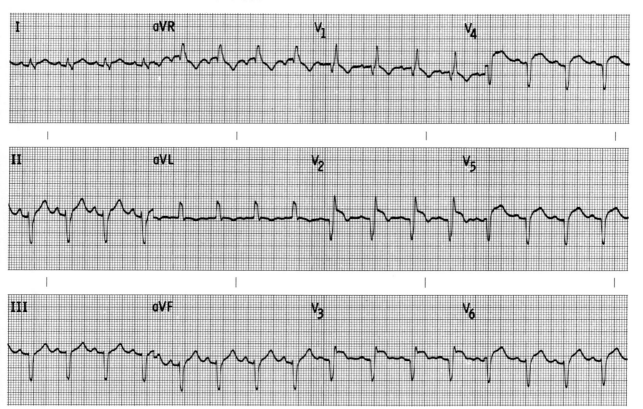

Case 24: Diagnosis

The cardiac rhythm is sinus with a rate of 98 beats per minute. It is easy to recognize evidences of acute extensive anterior MI (pathologic Q waves in leads V_{2-4} and embryonic r waves in leads V_1, V_5, and V_6 associated with marked S-T segment elevation and T wave inversion especially in leads V_{1-3}). In addition, there is a BFB which consists of RBBB and LAHB (QRS axis: -90 degrees). The P wave is slightly peaked in lead II suggestive of P-pulmonale.

The treatment of choice for acute BFB due to anterior MI is a prophylactic artificial cardiac pacing.

Case 25

This is a routine ECG tracing taken on an 89-year-old woman without any symptoms. She was found to be apparently healthy other than having mild systolic hypertension. She was not taking any drug.

1. *What is your ECG diagnosis?*
2. *What is the treatment of choice?*

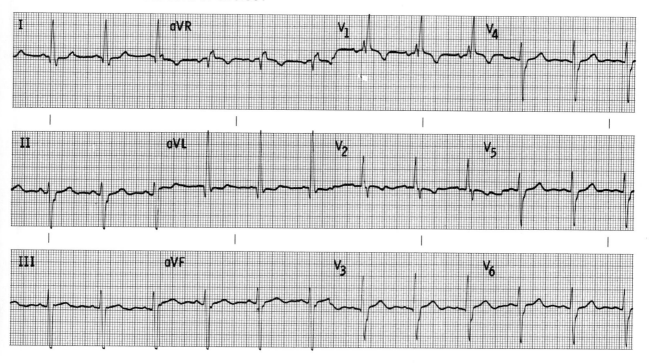

Case 25: Diagnosis

The cardiac rhythm is sinus with 72 beats per minute. The ECG abnormalities include BFB consisting of RBBB and LAHB (QRS axis: −60 degrees) and probable left ventricular hypertrophy as well as left atrial enlargement.

Chronic BFB needs no treatment as long as the patient is asymptomatic and there is no evidence of advanced BBBB (e.g., intermittent complete A-V block or Mobitz type II A-V block) confirmed by the Holter monitor ECG. Needless to say, BFB is a form of incomplete BBBB (see Case 23).

Case 26

This ECG tracing was taken on a 64-year-old man with coronary artery disease. He had been taking no medication other than intermittent sublingual nitroglycerin for chest pain.

1. *What is your ECG diagnosis?*
2. *Is an artificial pacemaker indicated?*

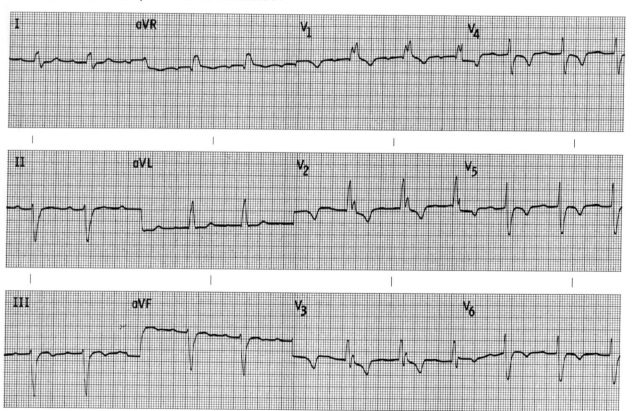

Case 26: Diagnosis

The cardiac rhythm is sinus (rate: 70 beats per minute) with first degree A-V block (P-R interval: 0.26 second). The diagnosis of BFB can be made without any difficulty on the basis of RBBB and LAHB (QRS axis: −80 degrees). Partial (incomplete) trifascicular block (TFB) is suspected because of a combination of first degree A-V block and BFB (see Case 23).

Another ECG abnormality is inverted T waves involving all precordial leads indicative of diffuse anterior MI.

Prophylactic artificial pacing is *not* indicated in this case as long as the patient has no symptoms (e.g., dizziness, syncope, or near-syncope) due to bradyarrhythmias (e.g., complete A-V block or Mobitz type II A-V block) as manifestation(s) of advanced BBBB (see Case 23). BFB or TFB usually does *not* occur as a result of angina pectoris. Acute BFB or TFB is nearly always due to acute anterior MI (see Cases 23 and 24).

Case 27

This ECG tracing was obtained from a 40-year-old man with idiopathic cardiomyopathy. He was not taking any drug.

1. *What is your ECG diagnosis?*
2. *Is artificial pacing indicated?*

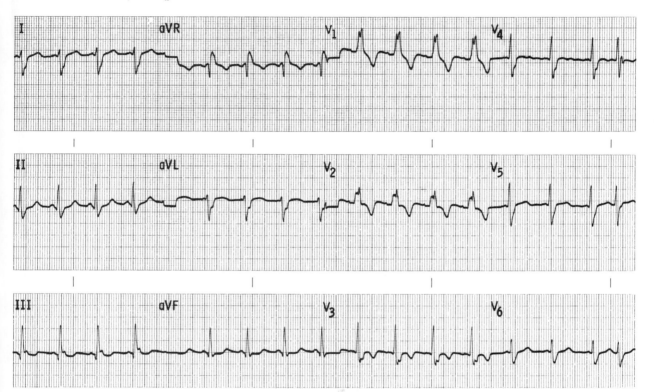

Case 27: Diagnosis

The cardiac rhythm is sinus (rate: 98 beats per minute) with an atrial premature contraction (APC) (the last beat). The obvious ECG abnormality is BFB which consists of RBBB and LPHB (the QRS axis: +130 degrees). It has been shown that a combination of RBBB and LPHB is commonly encountered in patients with idiopathic cardiomyopathy. Of course, BFB is a partial (incomplete) BBBB (see Case 23).

Artificial pacemaker is *not* indicated as long as there is no evidence of more advanced form of BBBB, such as intermittent Mobitz type II A-V block or complete A-V block (see Case 23).

In general, LPHB is much less common than LAHB because of two major reasons; namely, left posterior fascicle receives a dual blood supply in addition to having a deeper anatomical structure than left anterior fascicle. LPHB is uncommon either as an isolated finding or as a combination with RBBB.

By and large, it is impossible to predict when these patients with BFB (either a combination of RBBB and LAHB or a combination of RBBB and LPHB) eventually will develop a more advanced form of BBBB, even by using electrophysiologic study (e.g., determination of the H-V interval). It has been demonstrated that the mortality rate among individuals with asymptomatic chronic BFB has not been altered by the prophylactic artificial pacing even in the presence of markedly prolonged H-V interval (the interval from the His bundle potential to the ventricular deflection on the His bundle electrocardiogram) more than 70 milliseconds.

Case 28

A 70-year-old woman was brought to the emergency room because of rapid heart rate associated with marked weakness and shortness of breath. She was not taking any medication.

1. *What is your ECG diagnosis?*
2. *What is the treatment of choice?*
3. *Is artificial pacing indicated?*

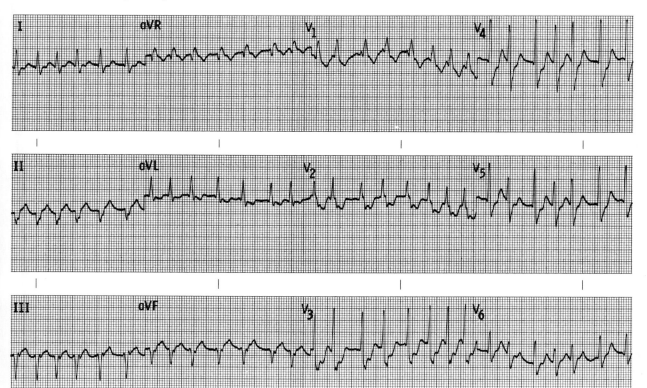

Case 28: Diagnosis

The cardiac rhythm is atrial fibrillation (AF) with very rapid ventricular response (rate: 170–200 per minute). Other ECG abnormality is BFB consisting of RBBB and LAHB (the QRS axis; −65 degrees). By superficial examination, ventricular tachycardia is closely simulated because of rapid ventricular rate with bizarre QRS complexes.

The treatment of choice for paroxysmal AF with rapid ventricular response is rapid (preferably intravenous injection) digitalization. When the clinical situation is extremely urgent and hemodynamic abnormality is pronounced (e.g., hypotension and/or acute pulmonary edema as a result of AF with very rapid ventricular rate), immediate application of direct current (DC) shock will be the treatment of choice. Many patients will require a maintenance oral digitalization even after restoration of sinus rhythm by DC shock or intravenous digitalization.

Artificial cardiac pacing is *not* indicated in this circumstance.

Case 29

A 51-year-old man visited the cardiac clinic because of rapid heart action a few hours in duration. He was not taking any drugs.

1. *What is the cardiac rhythm diagnosis?*
2. *What is the treatment of choice?*

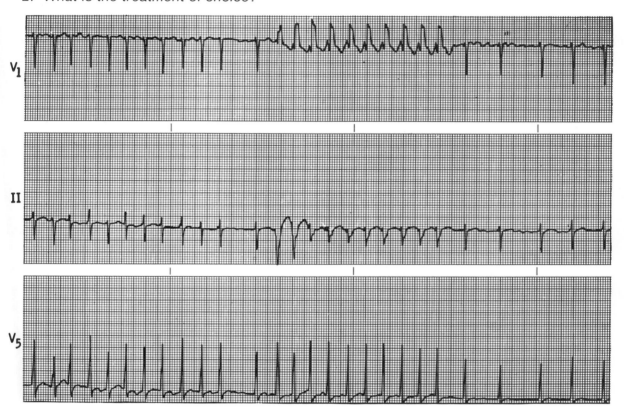

Case 29: Diagnosis

The cardiac rhythm is AF with a very rapid ventricular response (rate: 120–200 beats per minute) and frequent aberrant ventricular conduction (AVC). A consecutively occurring AVC closely mimics paroxysmal ventricular tachycardia (VT).

The diagnosis of VT is definitely excluded on the basis of the absence of postectopic pause and the presence of Ashman's phenomenon. Note the long ventricular cycle (R-R interval) immediately preceding the coupling interval (Ashman's phenomenon).

Ashman's phenomenon was first described by Ashman in 1945, and it is the most common cause of AVC. Ashman's phenomenon is best described as follows: *The longer the ventricular cycle, the longer the refractory period following it*; *the shorter the ventricular cycle, the shorter the refractory period.*

Various ECG findings to support AVC are summarized as follows:

ECG Findings to Support Aberrant Ventricular Conduction
(1) Ashman's phenomenon
(2) Bizarre QRS preceded by ectopic P wave
(3) No pause following bizarre beat(s), particularly in AF
(4) Irregular R-R cycle during consecutive AVC in AF or multifocal atrial tachycardia (MAT)
(5) Very short coupling interval in supraventricular premature beat (e.g., atrial premature contraction, APC).
(6) Extremely rapid ventricular rate in supraventricular tachyarrhythmias
(7) RBBB pattern
(8) Identical initial vector

In 80 to 85% of the cases, the AVC exhibits a RBBB *pattern.* In the remaining 15–20%, aberrantly conducted beats may demonstrate a LBBB *pattern*, or a LAHB or LPHB *pattern.* At times, AVC shows a BFB (a combination of a LAHB or LPHB and a RBBB) *pattern*, which is *functional* BFB.

The treatment of choice is rapid digitalization in this case.

It should be noted that the bizarre and broad QRS complexes due to AVC represent *functional* bundle branch block (left or right) and not *true* or *anatomical* bundle branch block.

Case 30

This ECG tracing was obtained from a 58-year-old man with coronary artery disease. He was not taking any medication.

1. *What is your ECG diagnosis?*
2. *Is an artificial pacemaker indicated?*

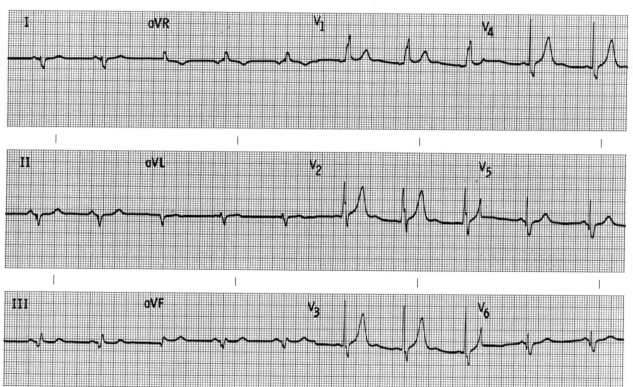

Case 30: Diagnosis

The cardiac rhythm is sinus with a rate of 60 beats per minute. The diagnosis of RBBB can be made without any difficulty. In addition, one can recognize readily the presence of diaphragmatic-lateral MI. Note pathologic Q waves or Q-S waves in leads I, II, III, and V_{5-6}. However, posterior MI may not be recognized easily by inexperienced readers. The diagnosis of posterior MI can be made on the basis of tall R waves in leads V_{1-3} with relatively tall T waves. The tall T waves in leads V_{1-3} due to posterior MI are obviously a reciprocal change—meaning deeply inverted T waves when using posterior ECG leads. Remember that a pure RBBB causes inverted or biphasic T waves in leads V_{1-3} with S-T segment depression.

Thus, the complete ECG diagnosis on this tracing is diaphragmatic-posterolateral MI (age undetermined) associated with RBBB. This patient had suffered from MI 2 months previously and his recovery was uneventful. In a review of his previous ECG tracings, RBBB was found to be the pre-existing ECG abnormality.

Artificial pacing is *not* indicated in this case. RBBB or LBBB of acute onset almost always occurs as a result of acute anteroseptal MI (see Cases 23 and 24).

Case 31

These ECG rhythm strips were obtained from an 84-year-old man who complained of dizziness and near-syncope associated with very slow pulse rate. He was not taking any drug.

1. *What is your ECG diagnosis?*
2. *What is the treatment of choice?*

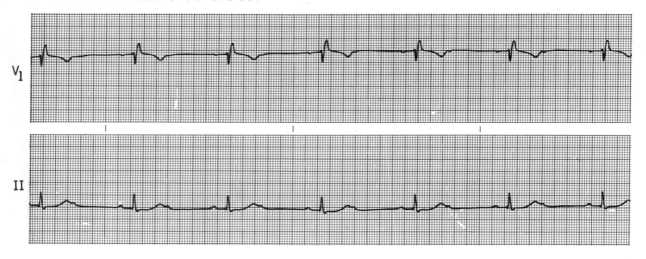

Case 31: Diagnosis

The cardiac rhythm is sinus (atrial rate: 80 beats per minutes) with 2:1 A-V block producing slow ventricular rate (rate: 40 beats per minuute). Note that every other P waves are not conducted to the ventricles. On superficial examination, marked sinus bradycardia is closely simulated when every other block sinus P waves (superimposed to the T waves) are not recognized.

Although the exact type of A-V block (Mobitz type I vs. Mobitz type II) can not be determined when dealing with 2:1 A-V block, a variant of Mobitz type II A-V block is almost certain when the QRS complexes show either RBBB or LBBB. In this case, the site of the block is below the A-V node meaning infranodal block (see Chapter 3).

Infranodal block is usually irreversible, and implantation of permanent pacemaker is the treatment of choice. Chronic Mobitz type II A-V block is considered to be due to a degenerative-sclerotic change in the conduction system, whereas acute Mobitz type II A-V block is nearly always produced by acute anteroseptal MI (see Chapter 3).

Case 32

These cardiac rhythm strips were obtained from a 64-year-old man with an artificial pacemaker.

1. *What is the ECG diagnosis?*
2. *What is the mode of artificial pacing?*

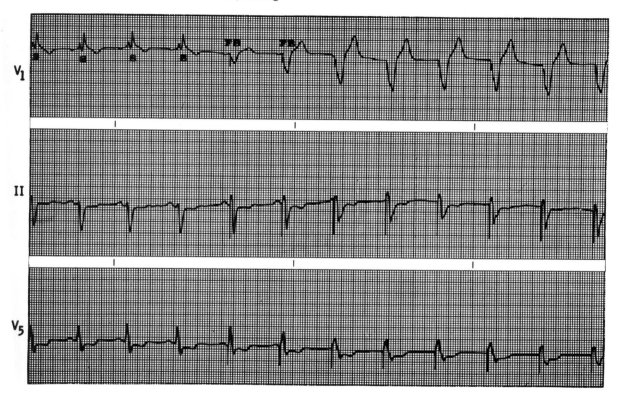

Case 32: Diagnosis

The underlying rhythm is sinus (S) with a rate of 75 beats per minute. The diagnosis of BFB, which consists of a RBBB and a LAHB, is easily made. An artificial pacemaker takes over the ventricular activity whenever the basic cardiac rhythm slows below the preset pacing rate. This is a characteristic feature of of the demand ventricular pacemaker.

The cardiac rhythm disorder before implantation of the artificial pacemaker was a Mobitz type II A-V block (see Chapter 3). Note the constant P-R intervals in all conducted sinus beats (S) until the blocked P waves occur. Thus, this patient demonstrates a combination of a BFB, consisting of RBBB and LAHB, and a Mobitz type II A-V block, an incomplete TFB. Note the occasional ventricular fusion beats (FB).

Case 33

This ECG tracing was taken on a 70-year-old man with mild congestive heart failure.

1. *What is your ECG diagnosis?*
2. *What drug is most likely responsible for producing this ECG abnormality?*

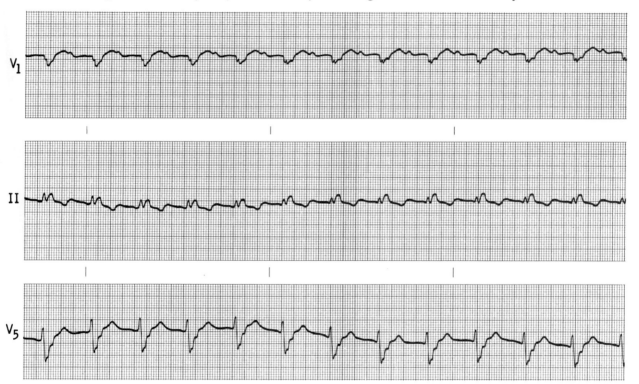

Case 33: Diagnosis

At a glance, the cardiac rhythm appears to be sinus rhythm with first degree A-V block. However, the actual heart rhythm diagnosis is atrial flutter (atrial rate: 156 beats per minute) with 2:1 A-V response. The characteristic sawtooth appearance of the atrial flutter waves is well demonstrated in lead II.

The atrial flutter rate is much slower than the usual in this case because of quinidine toxicity. In addition, the QRS complexes are very broad, again as a result of quinidine toxicity. Quinidine-induced broad QRS complexes represent diffuse or nonspecific intraventricular block rather than LBBB or RBBB. In other words, diffuse intraventricular block under this circumstance indicates intramyocardial block rather than any localized block in the bundle branch system.

Quinidine often causes markedly slow atrial flutter cycle as seen in this case because the refractory period of the atria is prolonged by the drug. Furthermore, quinidine often enhances the A-V conduction so that atrial flutter with 1:1 A-V conduction may result (see Case 65). Thus, administration of quinidine alone without digitalis to the patient with atrial flutter with 2:1 A-V conduction (see Case 57) is rather hazardous. Remember that the usual atrial rate in a pure atrial flutter ranges from 250 to 350 beats per minute.

Procainamide (Pronestyl) and disopyramide (Norpace) possess the same electrophysiologic properties as quinidine. Therefore, the same precaution must be exercised when these antiarrhythmic agents are administered.

Case 34

These ECG rhythm strips were obtained from a newborn infant with irreversible renal failure resulting from a congenital kidney anomaly. The infant died shortly after this ECG tracing was recorded.

1. *What is your ECG diagnosis?*
2. *What electrolyte imbalance is responsible for the production of these ECG abnormalities?*

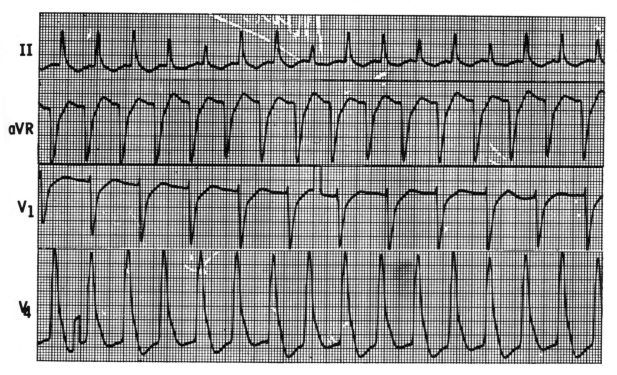

Case 34: Diagnosis

The P waves are not clearly visible because they show very low amplitude. The rhythm is sinus arrhythmia (the P waves are recognizable in lead I) with a rate of 95–125 beats per minute. The QRS complexes are very broad indicative of diffuse (nonspecific) intraventricular block.

The flat P waves with diffuse intraventricular block are characteristic features of far advanced hyperkalemia. It should be noted that peaking and tent-shaped T waves (the earliest change in hyperkalemia) may or may not be present in far advanced hyperkalemia. It is a well known fact that hyperkalemia is the most common electrolyte imbalance in renal failure.

The ECG finding in this tracing (flat P waves with broad QRS complex and relatively rapid heart rate) due to hyperkalemia closely simulates ventricular tachycardia.

Case 35

This ECG tracing was obtained from a 58-year-old man with chronic renal failure due to necrotizing glomerulonephritis proven by biopsy. He had been in the long-term hemodialysis program 3 times weekly for 18 months.

1. *What is your ECG diagnosis?*
2. *What electrolyte imbalance is responsible for the production of this ECG abnormality?*

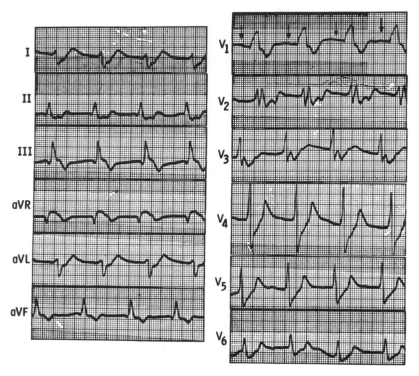

Case 35: Diagnosis

This electrocardiographic tracing was taken on admission. It shows flat P waves (indicated by arrows) BFB consisting of RBBB and LPHB (the QRS axis: +120 degrees) and peaked T waves due to marked hyperkalemia.

Laboratory findings included a hemoglobin level of 7.7 mg./100 ml., blood urea nitrogen 104 mg., sodium 143 mEq./L, potassium 9.0 mEq./L, chloride 108 mEq./L, carbon dioxide 13 mEq./L, calcium 4.2 mEq./L. Chest film showed a marked cardiomegaly with bilateral pleural effusion. Within 5 hours after hemodialysis, all of the aforementioned electrocardiographic abnormalities due to hyperkalemia disappeared.

Initial therapy consisted of intravenous injections of 50 cc. of 50 percent glucose, 10 units insulin, 1 ampule bicarbonate, 1 ampule calcium chloride and Kayexalate enema. He was hemodialyzed within 2 hours of admission to the CCU with a lowering of the serum potassium level to 4.2 mEq./L from the admission value of 9.0 mEq./L, 5 hours after admission. The patient was discharged 2 days after admission, fully recovered.

chapter 3

Atrioventricular Conduction Disturbance

Case 36

This ECG tracing was obtained from a 76-year-old woman with congestive heart failure due to mild hypertension. She had been taking hydrochlorothiazide 50 mg. every other day.

1. *What is your ECG diagnosis?*
2. *What is the treatment of choice for this cardiac arrhythmia?*

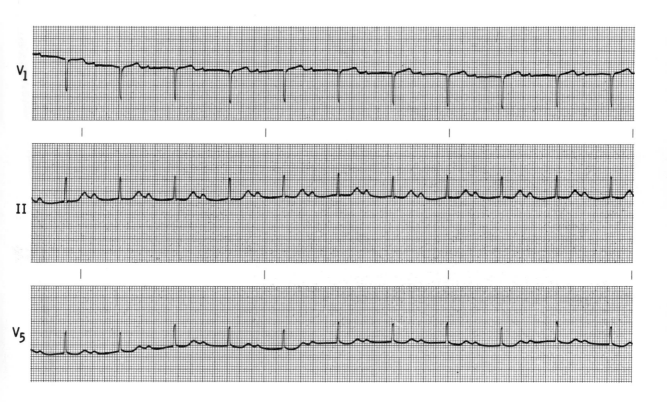

Case 36: Diagnosis

The cardiac rhythm is sinus (rate: 68 beats per minute) with first degree A-V block. Note that the P-R interval is markedly prolonged (P-R interval: 0.44 second) so that the P-R interval and the Q-T interval are almost identical. Other ECG abnormalities include left atrial enlargement and nonspecific S-T segment change.

No treatment is indicated for first degree A-V block.

Case 37

This ECG tracing was taken on a 79-year-old woman with coronary artery disease associated with moderate hypertension. She was admitted to the coronary care unit because of chest pain 2 days in duration. No medication was taken before admission.

1. *What is your ECG diagnosis?*
2. *What is the electrophysiologic mechanism that produces this cardiac arrhythmia?*
3. *Is an artificial pacemaker indicated?*

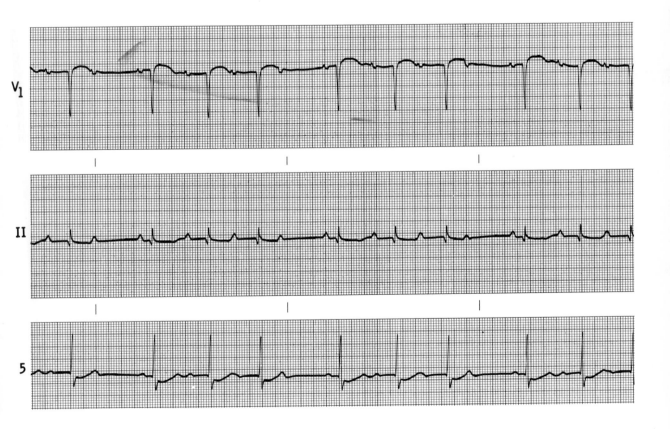

Case 37: Diagnosis

The cardiac rhythm is sinus (atrial rate: 83 beats per minute) with 4:3 Wenckebach (Mobitz type I) A-V block. The diagnosis of recent diaphragmatic (inferior) myocardial infarction (MI) can be made (only lead II is shown in this tracing). In addition, left atrial enlargement and left ventricular hypertrophy can be diagnosed without any difficulty.

The term "4:3" Wenckebach A-V block is used when every P wave is not conducted to the ventricles. In other words, three out of four P waves are conducted to the ventricles in this case. Note progressive lengthening of the P-R intervals until a blocked P wave occurs. In addition, the ventricular cycles (the R-R intervals) are progressively shortened until a ventricular pause (containing a blocked P wave) occurs. The long R-R interval is shorter than 2 P-P cycles.

The fundamental mechanism responsible for Wenckebach A-V block is diagrammatically illustrated in this page. The numbers represent hundredths of a second. The numbers in the upper row represent the atrial cycle (P-P interval) with a rate of 60 beats per minute. The numbers within the oblique lines at the A-V level indicate the A-V conduction time (P-R interval). The progressive lengthening of the P-R intervals is apparent until a blocked atrial impulse (dropped P wave) occurs. Following this blocked atrial impulse, the P-R interval shortens to its original value (0.20 second), and the sequence is repeated. The numbers in the lower row represent the duration of successive ventricular cycles. The progressive shortening of the ventricular cycle length (R-R interval) is due to the progressive increment of A-V conduction before the blocked atrial impulse and the decrement immediately following the blocked P wave. The numbers in parentheses in the lower row indicate the degree of increment or decrement in the ventricular cycle length.

Wenckebach A-V block is relatively common in recent diaphragmatic MI, and the A-V block is usually transient and self-limited. Thus, artificial pacing is *not* indicated under this circumstance as long as the patient is asymptomatic (as a result of the A-V block itself) and there is no hemodynamic abnormality. Wenckebach A-V block represents A-V nodal block (a block is in the A-V node).

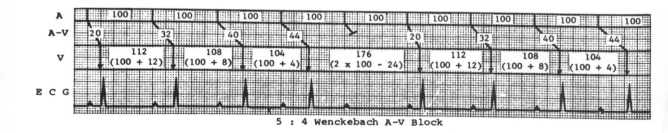

5 : 4 Wenckebach A-V Block

Case 38

These ECG rhythm strips were taken on a 67-year-old man with several episodes of near-syncope or syncope. He was not taking any medication.

1. *What is your ECG diagnosis?*
2. *Is an artificial pacemaker indicated?*

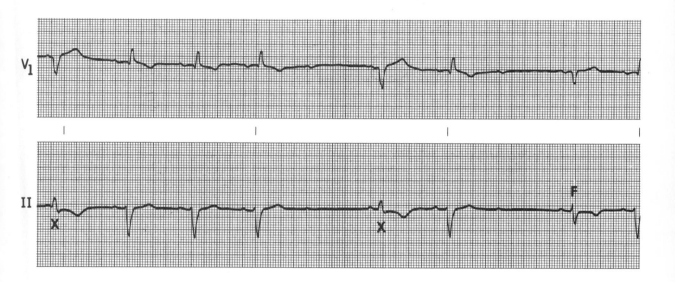

Case 38: Diagnosis

The cardiac rhythm is sinus (atrial rate: 60 beats per minute) with Mobitz type II A-V block and occasional ventricular escape beats (marked X) with one ventricular fusion beat (marked F). It is easy to recognize a bifascicular block (BFB) consisting of right bundle branch block (RBBB) and left anterior hemiblock (LAHB) (the QRS axis is estimated to be + 60 degrees).

It has been repeatedly stressed that Mobitz type II A-V block represents infranodal block which is a manifestation of incomplete bilateral bundle branch block (BBBB) [incomplete trifasicular block (TFB)—see Case 23]. Failure of the expected A-V junctional escape beat to appear following a long ventricular pause due to Mobitz type II A-V block supports the evidence of infranodal block. Again, the QRS complexes of all conducted beats in Mobitz type II A-V block almost always disclose either RBBB or left bundle branch block (LBBB), and at times BFB, as shown in this ECG tracing. Note constant P-R intervals in all conducted beats—a characteristic feature of Mobitz type II A-V block.

Every patient with Mobitz type II A-V block requires a permanent artificial pacemaker, since the A-V block is irreversible under this circumstance, even if asymptomatic.

Case 39

This ECG tracing was recorded from a 79-year-old man with a recent heart attack. He was not taking any medication before this admission to the coronary care unit.

1. *What is your ECG rhythm diagnosis?*
2. *Is an artificial pacemaker indicated?*

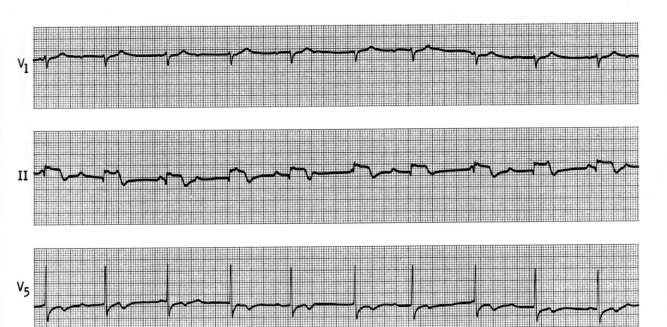

Case 39: Diagnosis

The cardiac rhythm is sinus (atrial rate: 95 beats per minute) with advanced (high degree) A-V block causing intermittent A-V junctional escape rhythm (ventricular rate: 58 beats per minute). Note that all QRS complexes are normal (narrow). There are occasional ventricular capture beats (conducted sinus beats—the 2nd, 5th, 7th, and 9th beats).

Obviously, this patient has suffered from acute diaphragmatic (inferior) MI (evidence of acute MI are shown in lead II—S-T segment elevation with inverted T wave and abnormal Q wave). A-V block of any degree in acute diaphragmatic MI represents A-V nodal block (a block in the A-V node), which is usually a reversible phenomenon.

An artificial pacemaker is *not* indicated as long as the patient is asymptomatic (no history of dizziness, syncope, or near syncope) without any hemodynamic abnormality (e.g., hypotension) from A-V block itself. As a rule, A-V block of any degree (even complete A-V block) in acute diaphragmatic MI is transient phenomenon and self-limited.

The T waves are inverted in lead V_5 and upright in lead V_1, and this finding indicates posterolateral myocardial ischemia—common coexisting abnormality associated with acute diaphragmatic MI.

Case 40

This ECG tracing (tracing A, shown on this page) and a second ECG taken at another time (1 hour apart) on the same day (tracing B, shown on the next page) were obtained from a 65-year-old man with fainting episodes. He was not taking any medication.

1. *What is your ECG diagnosis on both tracings?*
2. *What is the treatment of choice?*

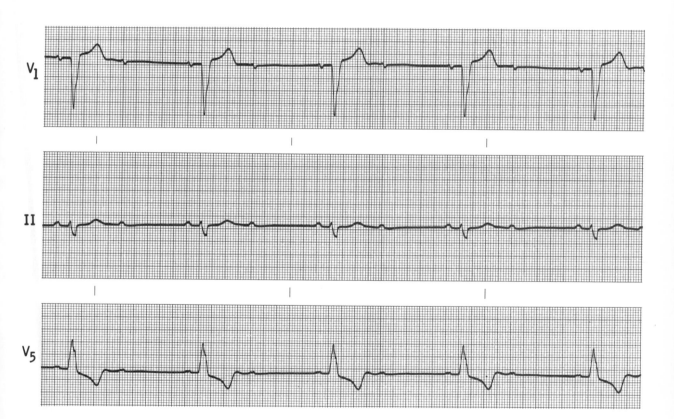

Case 40: Diagnosis

Tracing A: The cardiac rhythm is sinus (atrial rate: 60 beats per minute) with 2:1 A-V block (ventricular rate: 30 beats per minute) and LBBB. It is *not* 100% certain whether 2:1 A-V block in this tracing is a variant of Mobitz type II A-V block, although the probability of Mobitz type II A-V block is very high judging from the fact that the QRS complexes show LBBB. However, 2:1 A-V block in this ECG tracing has been proven to be unequivocally a variant of Mobitz type II A-V block, because another ECG (tracing B) taken 1 hour later demonstrates a characteristic feature of Mobitz type II A-V block.

Another interesting finding in this tracing is ventriculophasic sinus arrhythmia. That is, the P-P interval which includes the QRS complex is shorter than the P-P interval without QRS complex. Ventriculophasic sinus arrhythmia may be associated with other cardiac arrhythmias including complete A-V block and ventricular premature contraction (VPC). In the latter case, the P-P interval containing a VPC is shorter than the P-P interval without a VPC during a postectopic pause. The exact cause of ventriculophasic sinus arrhythmia is not clearly understood.

Tracing B: One hour later, the cardiac rhythm shows a typical Mobitz type II A-V block and LBBB. Note that all conducted beats show constant P-R intervals. Left atrial enlargement is suggested.

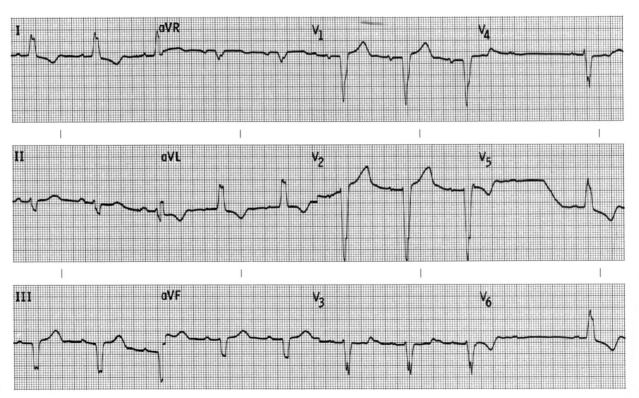

Treatment: Of course, the treatment of choice in this case is implantation of a permanent artificial pacemaker. Remember that Mobitz type II A-V block represents infranodal block—incomplete BBBB (incomplete TFB; see Case 23), and the block is irreversible. The P-R intervals of all conducted beats are slightly prolonged (P-R interval 0.24 second).

Case 41

A 74-year-old man was referred to a cardiologist for the evaluation of several episodes of near-syncope and dizziness. He was not taking any medication.

1. *What is your ECG diagnosis?*
2. *Is an artificial pacemaker indicated?*

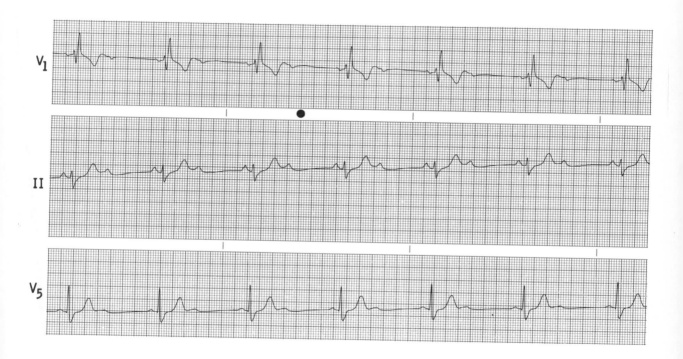

Case 41: Diagnosis

The cardiac rhythm is sinus (atrial rate: 84 beats per minute) with 2:1 A-V block (ventricular rate: 42 beats per minute) and a BFB consisting of RBBB and LAHB (the QRS axis is estimated to be −45 degrees). The 2:1 A-V block in this case is most likely a variant of Mobitz type II A-V block in view of coexisting BFB.

In addition, there is ventriculophasic sinus arrhythmia. Note that the R-R interval with a QRS complex is shorter than the R-R interval without QRS complex (see Case 40). The presence of ventriculophasic sinus arrhythmia is insignificant clinically.

The treatment of choice, needless to say, is permanent artificial pacemaker implantation.

Case 42

This ECG tracing was obtained from a 70-year-old man with frequent episodes of dizziness associated with slow pulse rate and mild congestive heart failure. He was not taking any medication and there was no history of chest pain.

1. *What is your ECG diagnosis?*
2. *What most likely is the underlying disease process in his heart?*
3. *What is the treatment of choice?*

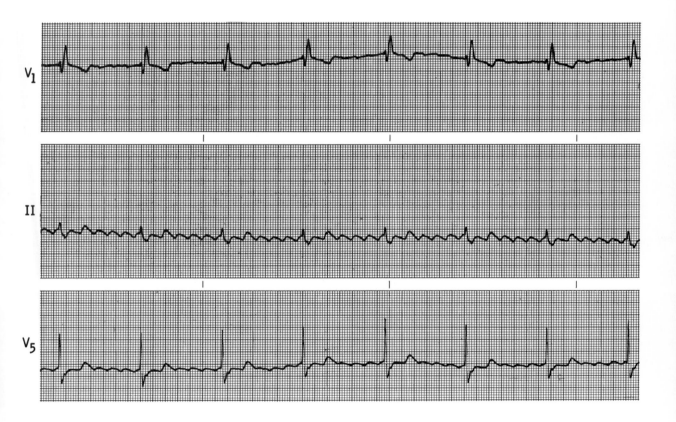

Case 42: Diagnosis

The underlying rhythm is atrial flutter (atrial rate: 282 beats per minute) with 6:1 A-V block (ventricular rate: 47 beats per minute) and a BFB consisting of RBBB and LAHB (the QRS axis is estimated to be −50 degrees). It is rather uncommon to observe 5:1 or 6:1 A-V block in atrial flutter. In most cases, A-V junctional or ventricular escape rhythm takes over the ventricular activity in advanced (5:1 or higher) A-V block in atrial flutter.

The A-V block in this case most likely represents infranodal A-V block, judging from the QRS complex morphology—BFB. In addition, sick sinus syndrome (SSS) is most likely responsible for the production of chronic atrial flutter with advanced A-V block (see Case 1). It can be said that a degenerative-sclerotic process in the sinus node as well as the entire conduction system produced the diffuse conduction abnormality and the sinus node dysfunction (see Case 1).

The treatment of choice is permanent artificial pacemaker implantation (see Case 2).

Case 43

This ECG tracing was obtained from a 41-year-old man with cardiomyopathy associated with several episodes of near-syncope. He was not taking any drug.

1. *What is your ECG diagnosis?*
2. *What is the treatment of choice?*

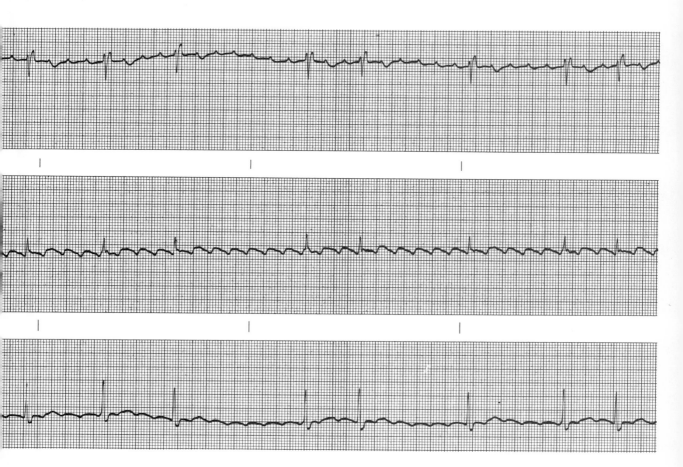

Case 43: Diagnosis

The cardiac rhythm is atrial flutter (atrial rate: 240 beats per minute) with advanced (varying degree) A-V block producing a very slow (ventricular rate: 35–45 beats per minute) and irregular ventricular cycle. This ECG finding is most likely a late manifestation of SSS. In addition, the diagnosis of RBBB can be made without any difficulty. The diagnostic criteria and various ECG manifestations of SSS have been described in detail previously (see Cases 1 and 4). RBBB or LBBB often coexists with SSS.

Permanent artificial pacemaker is indicated in this patient (see Case 2). The atrial flutter cycle is slightly slower than usual in this case, and the finding is not uncommon in patients with idiopathic cardiomyopathy. Remember that the usual atrial flutter cycle ranges from 250 to 350 beats per minute.

Case 44

This ECG tracing was recorded from an 80-year-old woman with Adams-Stokes syndrome. She had fainted on several occasions, but was not taking any medication before this admission to the intermediate coronary care unit.

1. *What is your ECG diagnosis?*
2. *Is an artificial pacemaker indicated?*

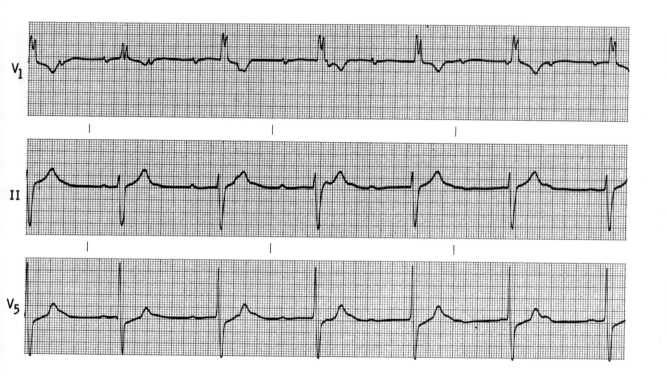

Case 44: Diagnosis

The cardiac rhythm is sinus (atrial rate: 83 beats per minute), with complete A-V block producing ventricular escape (idioventricular) rhythm (rate: 38 beats per minute). It should be noted that the QRS complexes are broad and bizarre, and there is no relationship between the P waves and the QRS complexes—meaning complete A-V dissociation.

The site of the complete A-V block in this case is, needless to say, in the bundle branch system. Thus, complete A-V block represents infra-His block—meaning complete BBBB or complete TFB (see Case 23). Of course, complete BBBB is irreversible.

The treatment of choice is unquestionably a permanent artificial pacemaker implantation. When a cardiac surgeon is not immediately available for the implantation, a temporary artificial pacemaker should be inserted by a cardiologist immediately until the surgeon becomes available.

Case 45

Digitalis intoxication was diagnosed in a 77-year-old man with hypertensive heart disease on the basis of marked slowing of the heart rate associated with worsening of congestive heart failure.

1. What is your cardiac rhythm diagnosis?
2. Is artificial pacing indicated?

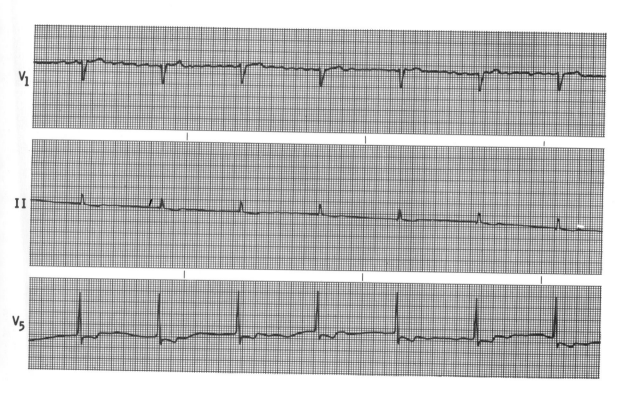

Case 45: Diagnosis

The underlying cardiac rhythm is atrial fibrillation, but the ventricular cycle is regular with slow ventricular rate. Thus, the rhythm diagnosis is atrial fibrillation with A-V junctional escape rhythm (ventricular rate: 45 beats per minute) due to complete A-V block (A-V nodal block) resulting in complete A-V dissociation.

Under this circumstance, two major factors, ventricular rate and presence or absence of symptom (e.g., fainting, dizziness, hypotension, etc.), will determine the indication or nonindication of the artificial pacing. In general, an artificial pacemaker is considered to be indicated when the ventricular rate in complete A-V block is slower than 45 beats per minute. An artificial pacemaker is definitely indicated for symptomatic complete A-V block. As a rule, the patient with complete A-V block is often symptomatic when the ventricular rate of the escape rhythm is slower than 45 beats per minute.

Needless to say, discontinuation of digitalis is the first and the most important therapeutic approach for the patient with digitalis intoxication.

Left ventricular hypertrophy is suspected, and prominent U waves are suggestive of hypokalemia. It is well documented that hypokalemia frequently predisposes to digitalis toxicity.

It should be remembered that digitalis-induced A-V block of any degree always represents A-V nodal block (a block in the A-V node), and A-V block is usually reversible upon discontinuation of digitalis.

Case 46

Tracing A (12-lead ECG shown on this page) and tracing B (exercise ECG test shown on the next page) were taken on a 35-year-old woman with known congenital complete A-V block. She was found to be asymptomatic, and there was no evidence of other coexisting cardiac anomaly.

1. *What is the main reason for performing the exercise ECG test in patients with congenital complete A-V block?*
2. *What is the usual expected functional capacity under this circumstance?*
3. *Does congenital complete A-V block usually represent A-V nodal block or infranodal block?*
4. *Is an artificial pacemaker indicated?*

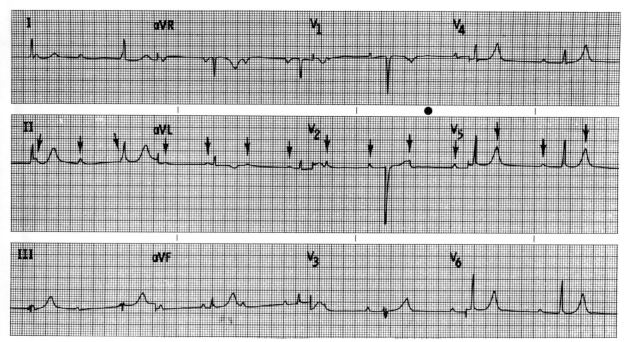

R.L., 35 F. – CONGENITAL A-V BLOCK (#1) RESTING ECG

Case 46: Diagnosis

Her resting 12-lead ECG (tracing A) shows sinus rhythm (indicated by arrows, atrial rate: 86 beats per minute) with A-V junctional escape rhythm (ventricular rate: 42 beats per minute) due to complete A-V block, and otherwise within normal limits.

Congenital complete A-V block usually represents A-V nodal block—yet the congenital A-V block is permanent.

Exercise ECG test is usually performed under this circumstance primarily in order to assess the functional capacity rather than the diagnosis of any possible coexisting heart disease. The functional capacity in most patients with congenital complete A-V block is estimated to be generally near normal or normal unless a coexisting cardiac anomaly is present.

The tracing B shown in this page is her exercise ECG. The strips A are resting ECG, whereas the strips B to G were recorded during exercise. The strips H and I represent postexercise ECG. Arrows indicate sinus P waves. The maximal atrial (sinus) rate reached 176 beats per minute, but the maximal ventricular rate was only 107 beats per minute. Complete A-V block persisted throughout the exercise ECG test as expected. Her functional capacity was considered to be normal, although she developed occasional

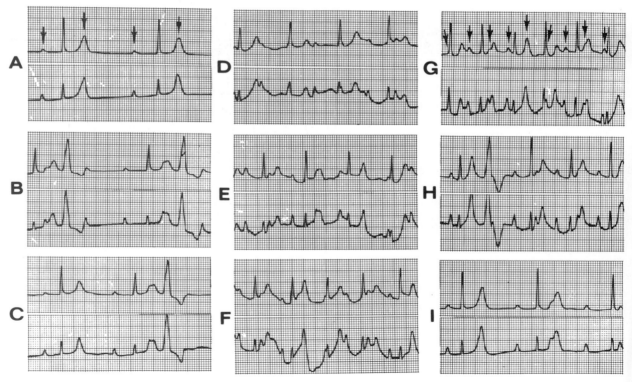

R.L., 35 F. - Congenital A-V block (#2) Exercise ECG Test

VPCs during exercise. In fact, VPCs are not uncommon in patients with congenital complete A-V block even at rest, but VPCs seldom cause any clinically significant consequences under this circumstance.

Permanent artificial pacemaker is recommended for all patients with congenital complete A-V block even if they are asymptomatic because of irreversible nature of the A-V block under this circumstance. In fact, most patients with congenital complete A-V block eventually become symptomatic as they get older unless paced.

chapter 4

Differential Diagnosis of Cardiac Arrhythmias

Case 47

This ECG tracing was obtained from a 20-year-old man with moderate hypertension. He denied any symptom, and the hypertension was considered to be essential (idiopathic). He was taking hydrochlorothiazide 50 mg. daily.

1. *What is your ECG diagnosis?*
2. *What is the treatment of choice?*

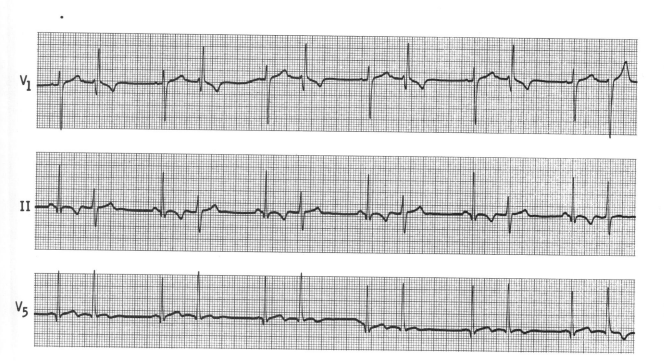

Case 47: Diagnosis

The underlying cardiac rhythm is sinus, but there are frequent atrial premature contractions (APCs) producing atrial bigeminy. The QRS complexes of APCs are bizarre, and they show predominantly right bundle branch block (RBBB) *pattern*. This finding is called aberrant ventricular conduction (AVC), which occurs when the cardiac impulse is conducted to the ventricles during their partial refractory period. Remember that AVC most frequently discloses RBBB *pattern* (up to 80–85% of cases), while left bundle branch block (LBBB) *pattern* due to AVC is rather uncommon. APCs with AVC closely resemble ventricular premature contractures (VPCs) when premature ectopic P waves are not recognized. In addition, the P-R interval of the APC is conducted in the A-V junction during its partial refractory period.

During atrial bigeminy, the QRS complexes of the APCs frequently show AVC as a result of the Ashman's phenomenon. The Ashman's phenomenon has been described in detail previously (see Case 29). Likewise, the P-R interval of the APC tends to be longer during atrial bigeminy, again as a result of the Ashman's phenomenon. Remember that the refractoriness of the heart beat is directly influenced by the preceding ventricular cycle (R-R interval).

By and large, no active treatment is indicated for APCs as long as there is no significant symptom (e.g., palpitations, chest discomfort, etc.) directly due to APCs. However, it is always wise to look for any possible cause for frequent APCs. For example, emotional tension, excessive use of coffee, tea, or cola drinks, heavy cigarette smoking, and electrolyte imbalance frequently cause APCs, VPCs, or other cardiac arrhythmias. When a direct cause responsible for the production of any arrhythmia is found, the causative factor should be eliminated or controlled. In addition, a small dosage (e.g., 10–20 mg., 3–4 times daily) of propranolol (Inderal) is usually effective under these circumstances.

The S-T segment and T wave abnormality with high left ventricular voltage indicates left ventricular hypertrophy.

Case 48

A 66-year-old mildly hypertensive woman was seen at the hypertensive clinic for evaluation of irregular heart rhythm. She was relatively asymptomatic except for occasional palpitations. She was not taking any medication.

1. *What is your ECG diagnosis?*
2. *What is the treatment of choice?*

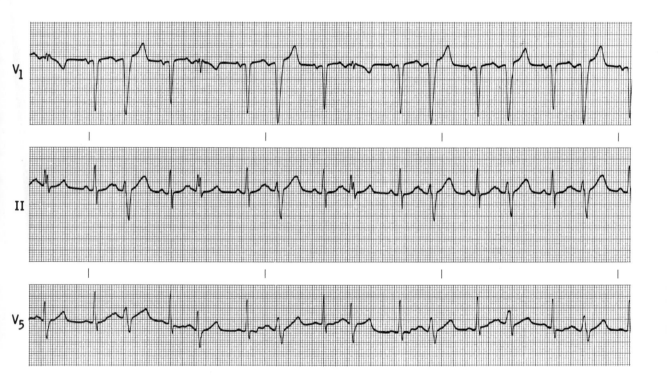

Case 48: Diagnosis

The underlying cardiac rhythm is sinus, but there are frequent APCs causing atrial bigeminy. The QRS complexes of APCs with AVC show a predominantly LBBB *pattern*, which is a rather uncommon occurrence. Remember that an RBBB *pattern* is observed much more frequently (up to 80–85%) during AVC (see Case 47). The basic reason why AVC is very common during atrial bigeminy has been fully described (see Cases 29 and 48).

When any direct cause (e.g., excessive use of coffee) for the production of APCs is not found, propranolol (Inderal) will be the drug of choice, because the drug will be effective for the arrhythmia as well as for hypertension.

This ECG tracing was obtained from a 42-year-old man with no known heart disease.

1. *What is your ECG diagnosis?*
2. *What is the treatment of choice?*

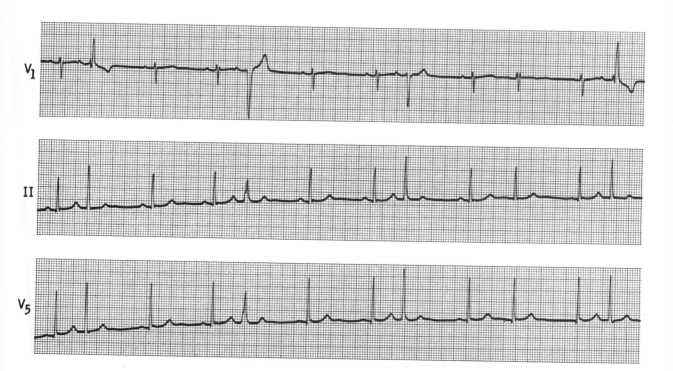

V₁

II

V₅

Case 49: Diagnosis

The underlying cardiac rhythm is sinus with a rate of 60 beats per minute. Note frequent APCs with aberrant ventricular conduction of varying degrees. The QRS complexes of the APCs showing AVC exhibit various configurations. That is, some APCs demonstrate RBBB *pattern* whereas others show LBBB *pattern*. It is also interesting to recognize that the APCs are originating at least from two different foci. For example, an APC (the 10th beat) discloses a different ectopic P wave configuration with a different coupling interval when one compares those findings with other APCs. Thus, this ECG tracing shows multifocal APCs with AVC of varying degrees. AVC occurs because the atrial premature impulse is conducted to the ventricles during their partial refractory period. Frequent APCs with AVC of varying contours closely simulate frequent multifocal VPCs.

As far as the therapeutic approach is concerned, any possible causative factor (e.g., excessive use of coffee, tea, or cola drinks, cigarette smoking, emotional stress, etc.) should be identified and eliminated (or controlled) if possible. In addition, common disorders which frequently produce a variety of cardiac arrhythmias should be investigated. For instance, mitral valve prolapse syndrome and hyperthyroidism should be ruled out because these disorders commonly produce various arrhythmias. Furthermore, cardiomyopathy or any other common heart diseases should be always investigated when dealing with persisting and unexplainable arrhythmia. Of course, a variety of arrhythmias may be encountered not uncommonly in apparently healthy individuals.

If the individual is found to be free of any known cardiac or noncardiac disorder, and if no possible underlying cause is found, no treatment is indicated as long as the APCs produce no significant symptom (e.g., palpitations, feeling of strange sensation, or skipped heart beats in the chest, etc.). When APCs are symptomatic, however, propranolol (Inderal) will be the drug of choice (10–20 mg., 3–4 times daily). Inderal is very effective for various cardiac arrhythmias in apparently healthy individuals as well as those with mitral valve prolapse syndrome or mild hyperthyroidism.

Case 50

These ECG rhythm strips were taken on a 71-year-old man with hypertensive heart disease. He was not taking any medication.

1. *What is your ECG diagnosis?*
2. *What is the treatment of choice?*

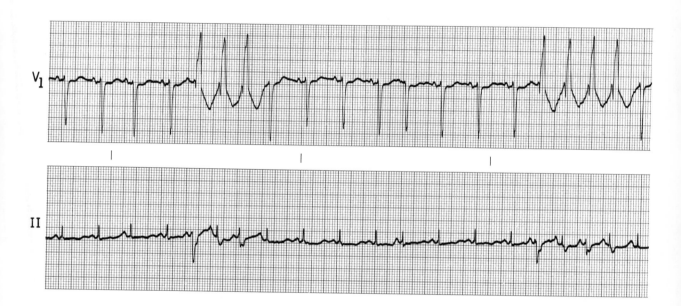

Case 50: Diagnosis

The underlying cardiac rhythm is sinus tachycardia with a rate of 103 beats per minute. There are frequent APCs, and some of them occur consecutively. When 2 or more ectopic beats occur consecutively, the term "group beats" or "grouped beats" is used. The term "atrial tachycardia" is used when 6 or more APCs occur consecutively. Thus, these cardiac rhythm strips demonstrated frequent atrial group beats (3–4 in-a-row). In addition, the APCs with group beats exhibit bizarre and broad QRS complexes as a result of AVC. Needless to say, frequent VPCs with group beats are closely simulated under this circumstance, but a premature P wave preceding each bizarre QRS complex (see lead II) excludes a possibility of VPCs.

The general therapeutic approach to APCs has been described previously (see Case 49). When frequent APCs produce significant symptom, propranolol should be tried first, providing there is no contraindication. Quinidine (0.3–0.4 g., 4 times daily) will be an alternative choice, especially when Inderal is found to be ineffective or contraindicated. No active treatment is indicated, however, when the individuals with APCs are totally asymptomatic.

Case 51

A 73-year-old man was evaluated at the cardiac clinic because of slow pulse rate. He was asymptomatic, however, and was not taking any medication.

1. *What is your ECG diagnosis?*
2. *What is the treatment of choice?*

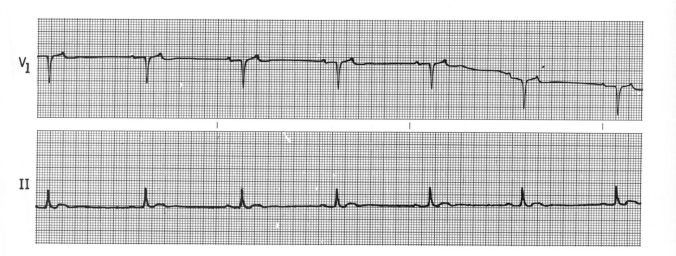

Case 51: Diagnosis

The underlying cardiac rhythm is sinus, but there are frequent nonconducted (blocked) APCs producing blocked atrial bigeminy. The blocked atrial premature P waves are superimposed on the early portion of the T waves of the preceding beats. Blocked or nonconducted APCs occur when the ectopic atrial impulse is conducted to the A-V junction during its absolute refractory period. By and large, a blocked atrial premature beat is observed when the coupling interval (the interval from the ectopic P wave to the basic sinus P wave of the preceding beat) is very short as seen in this ECG tracing. Otherwise, a blocked APC tends to occur when there is Ashman's phenomenon (see Case 29).

Blocked APCs superficially resemble many other cardiac arrhythmias including sinus bradycardia, sinus arrhythmia, 2:1 A-V block, sinus arrest, and sino-atrial block. When nonconducted APCs occur as a bigeminy (nonconducted or blocked atrial bigeminy) as shown in this ECG tracing, the finding closely simulates marked sinus bradycardia because the reader may not recognize all blocked ectopic P waves.

The therapeutic approach to the nonconducted (blocked) APCs is the same as that to the ordinary APCs (see Cases 47 and 49). Artificial cardiac pacing is *not* indicated.

Case 52

This ECG tracing was taken at a cardiologist's office for the evaluation of palpitations on a 59-year-old woman with chronic cor-pulmonale. She had been taking digoxin 0.25 mg. daily for several months, but there was no clinical sign of digitalis toxicity.

1. *What is your ECG diagnosis?*
2. *What is the treatment of choice?*

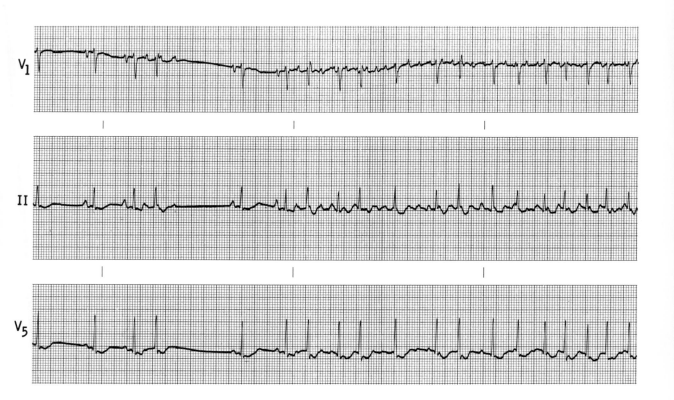

Case 52: Diagnosis

The underlying cardiac rhythm is sinus, but paroxysmal atrial flutter-fibrillation is initiated by frequent APCs. The term, "atrial flutter-fibrillation" is used when the atrial flutter cycle is *not* regular throughout and ill-defined in some areas—meaning a mixture of atrial flutter and fibrillation.

It has been well documented that various atrial tachyarrhythmias are common in patients with chronic cor-pulmonale, and multifocal atrial tachycardia (MAT) is particularly common under this circumstance (see Cases 54 and 64). Note peaking P waves of the sinus in origin indicative of P-pulmonale.

Various atrial tachyarrhythmias can be controlled or even eliminated when the underlying pulmonary disease is properly treated so that pulmonary functions improve. Otherwise, quinidine will be the drug of choice for paroxysmal atrial fibrillation (AF) or flutter-fibrillation when the patient is already taking digitalis. When digitalis is not used previously, however, digitalization should be carried out first before the use of quinidine. Digitalis alone may be able to terminate and prevent a variety of atrial tachyarrhythmias in many cases. Her serum digoxin level was found to be 1.2 ng./ml. (the normal therapeutic range: (1.0–2.5 ng./ml.). It should be pointed out that AF, flutter or flutter-fibrillation is extremely rare in digitalis intoxication (see Chapter 7).

A 36-year-old woman was referred to a cardiologist for evaluation of her palpitations. Her 12-lead ECG was within normal limits, but an echocardiogram confirmed a mitral valve prolapse syndrome (MVPS). She was not taking any drugs when the Holter monitor ECG was recorded.

1. *What is the cardiac rhythm diagnosis?*
2. *What is the treatment of choice?*

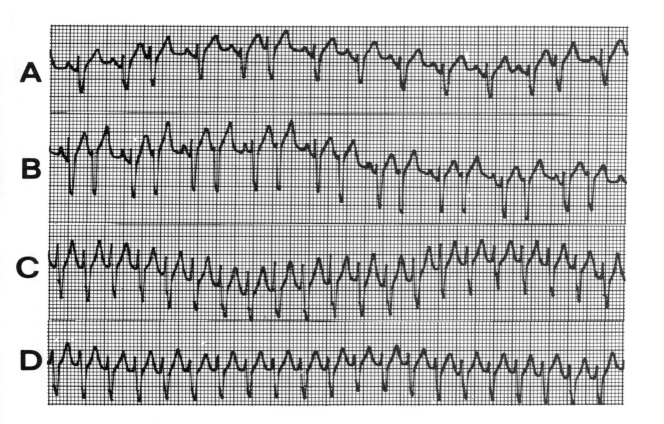

Case 53: Diagnosis

The rhythm strips A through D are not continuous. The underlying cardiac rhythm is sinus tachycardia (rate: 130 beats per minute). There are frequent APCs causing atrial bigeminy (strip B), which leads to paroxysmal atrial tachycardia (rate: 210 beats per minute, strips C and D).

It is a well known fact that various cardiac arrhythmias, particularly atrial tachyarrhythmias and VPCs are common in patients with MVPS. Under these circumstances, the drug of choice is oral propranolol (Inderal), 10–40 mg., 3–4 times daily.

Case 54

This ECG tracing was obtained from a 69-year-old man with mild congestive heart failure. He was examined at the cardiac clinic for the evaluation of his cardiac arrhythmia and the management of congestive heart failure. He was not taking any medication.

1. *What is your ECG diagnosis?*
2. *What is the most common underlying disorder responsible for the production of this arrhythmia?*
3. *What is the treatment of choice?*

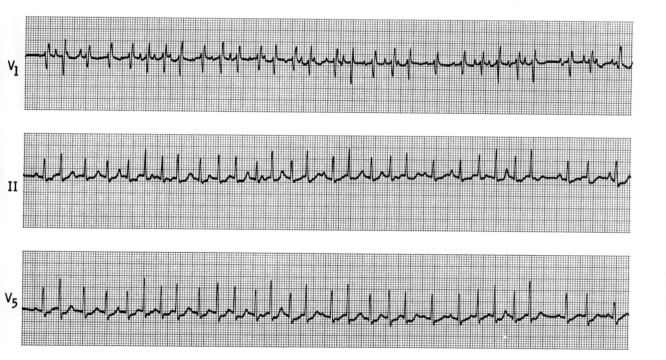

Case 54: Diagnosis

The cardiac rhythm is MAT with varying A-V response (atrial rate: 180–200 beats per minute) and occasional AVC.

The diagnostic criteria of MAT are as follows:

(a) Varying configurations of P waves
(b) Varying P-P cycles
(c) Varying P-R intervals with or without blocked P waves
(d) Atrial rate between 120 and 250 beats per minute (at times slower than 120 beats per minute)
(e) Isoelectric line between P waves
(f) Common occurrence of P-pulmonale

MAT closely simulates atrial fibrillation (AF). MAT has many other names including chaotic atrial rhythm, chaotic atrial tachycardia, malignant atrial tachycardia, wandering pacemaker in the atria, etc. Not uncommonly, MAT may be preceded by or followed by atrial fibrillation or flutter.

MAT is most commonly observed in patients with chronic cor-pulmonale (up to 75% of cases with all MAT found in chronic cor-pulmonale). Less commonly, MAT may be encountered in patients with pulmonary embolism, severe pneumonia, coronary artery disease, hypoxia due to various causes and digitalis toxicity.

The best therapeutic approach to MAT is to treat the underlying disorder, particularly chronic cor-pulmonale. If MAT persists and the ventricular rate is fast, as seen in this case, digitalis should be tried first, unless MAT is considered to be digitalis-induced. Unfortunately, digitalis alone does not terminate MAT in most cases. Rather, digitalis often causes slow ventricular rate by virtue of increased A-V block. Propranolol (Inderal) is found to be effective in some cases with MAT providing there is no contraindication. Otherwise, quinidine may be tried when MAT persists even after digitalization. By and large, MAT is difficult to treat with any antiarrhythmic agent with or without digitalization. Thus, the proper management of the underlying disorder responsible for the production of MAT is crucial.

In addition, there are evidences of incomplete RBBB and nonspecific abnormality of the S-T segment and T waves. Note peaking P waves indicative of P-pulmonale.

Case 55

This ECG tracing was obtained from a 70-year-old man who was admitted to the coronary care unit because of acute congestive heart failure and chest pain with several hours in duration. He was not taking any drug.

1. *What is your ECG diagnosis?*
2. *What is the treatment of choice?*

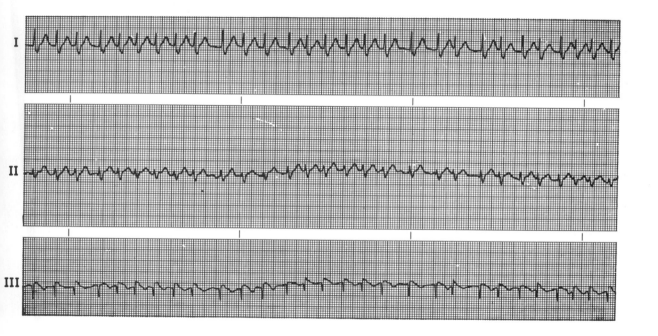

Case 55: Diagnosis

The cardiac rhythm shows AF associated with RBBB with a very rapid ventricular response (ventricular rate: 160–190 beats per minute). Note a deep and broad S wave in lead I indicating a delayed activation of the right ventricle as a result of RBBB. Thus, the diagnosis of RBBB can be made without having lead V_1. Needless to say, it will be easier to diagnose RBBB when lead V_1 is available—showing RR'. Ventricular tachycardia is closely simulated because of rapid ventricular rate and bizarre and broad QRS complexes. However, ventricular tachycardia is definitely excluded on the basis of a grossly irregular ventricular cycle.

The diagnosis of acute diaphragmatic myocardial infarction (MI) is made on the basis of pathologic Q waves in leads III and aVF with S-T segment elevation (lead aVF is not shown here).

The treatment of choice is rapid digitalization for AF with rapid ventricular response regardless of underlying disease. If the clinical picture is extremely urgent, however, direct current shock should be applied immediately before digitalization. Although there is a significant controversy regarding the use of digitalis in patients with acute MI, digitalis is usually effective for AF with rapid ventricular response even in the presence of acute MI.

Case 56

These cardiac rhythm strips were obtained from an 89-year-old woman with acute congestive heart failure due to hypertensive heart disease.

1. *What is the cardiac rhythm diagnosis?*
2. *What is the treatment of choice?*

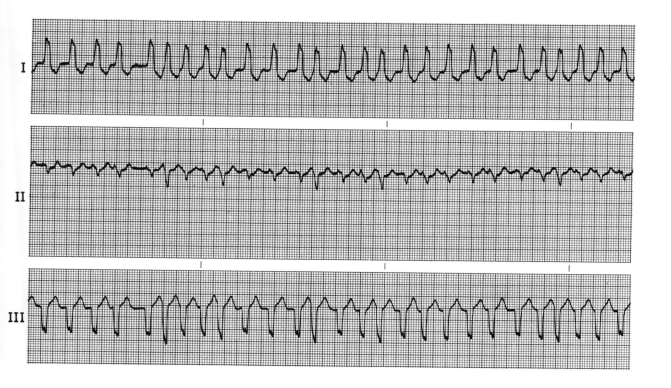

Case 56: Diagnosis

The cardiac rhythm shows AF associated with LBBB with a very rapid ventricular response (ventricular rate: 170–200 beats per minute). In the differential diagnosis, ventricular tachycardia, which is considered because of the rapid ventricular rate and bizarre and broad QRS complexes, is definitely excluded on the basis of a grossly irregular ventricular cycle. In elderly individuals, atrial fibrillatory waves are usually not clearly evident and this finding is termed "fine" AF to distinguish it from "coarse" AF (amplitude of the fibrillatory wave over 1 mm.).

As far as the underlying disease is concerned, a fine AF is usually due to a coronary and/or hypertensive heart disease, whereas a coarse AF is nearly always found in patients with rheumatic heart disease, and particularly in patients with mitral stenosis. Less commonly, a coarse AF may be found in patients with hyperthyroidism.

The patient was rapidly digitalized, with marked improvement.

Case 57

A 67-year-old man was found to have a very rapid heart rate associated with acute congestive heart failure. He was not taking any medication.

1. *What is your ECG diagnosis?*
2. *What is the treatment of choice?*

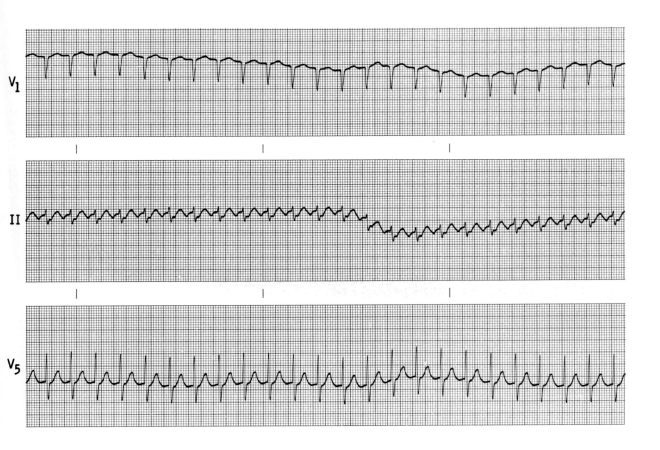

V₁

II

V₅

Case 57: Diagnosis

The cardiac rhythm is atrial flutter (atrial rate: 300 beats per minute) with 2:1 A-V conduction (ventricular rate: 150 beats per minute). Note that all other atrial flutter waves are not conducted to the ventricles because of a physiologic phenomenon—long refractory period in the A-V junction. Thus, under this circumstance, the term "2:1 A-V conduction" is used rather than "2:1 A-V block." Remember that A-V block means abnormally prolonged refractory period in the A-V conduction system. In other words, "2:1 A-V conduction" in atrial flutter is a normal physiologic phenomenon.

The usual atrial flutter cycle ranges from 250 to 350 beats per minute in a pure atrial flutter, and the ventricular rate is a half of the atrial rate. In general, a possibility of atrial flutter with 2:1 A-V conduction should always be considered when dealing with a regular tachycardia with ventricular rate around 150 beats per minute, especially when P waves are not discernible and the QRS complexes are normal.

The treatment of choice is rapid digitalization. When the clinical situation is extremely urgent, however, immediate application of direct current (DC) shock will be the treatment of choice.

There is left axis deviation of the QRS complexes (axis: −30 degrees).

Case 58

This ECG tracing was obtained from a 68-year-old woman with advanced congestive heart failure due to hypertensive heart disease.

    1. *What is your ECG diagnosis?*
    2. *What is the treatment of choice?*

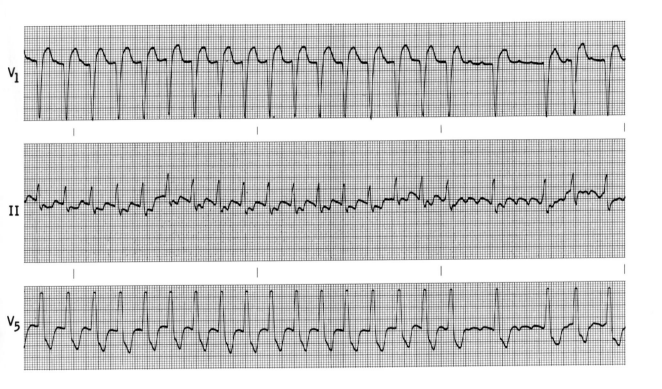

Case 58: Diagnosis

The cardiac rhythm is atrial flutter (atrial rate: 300 beats per minute) with predominantly 2:1 A-V response. The atrial flutter cycle is clearly visible during slower ventricular rate (the last portion of the tracing). Because of broad QRS complexes as a result of LBBB, ventricular tachycardia is closely simulated.

The patient has improved markedly after digitalization.

LBBB is most commonly found in patients with hypertensive heart disease.

Case 59

A 62-year-old man with coronary artery disease was seen at the cardiac clinic for a follow-up visit after recovery from a heart attack 6 months previously. He denied any chest pain, dizziness, or near-syncope, but he had experienced slight shortness of breath on exertion in the past several months. He was not taking any medication other than aspirin—2 tablets per day.

1. *What is your ECG diagnosis?*
2. *Is an artificial pacing indicated?*

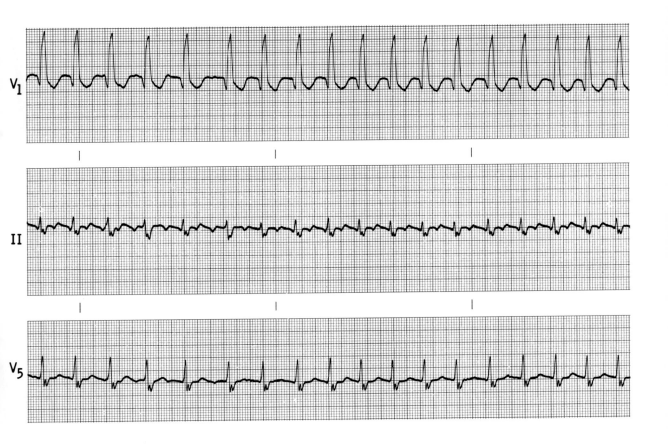

Case 59: Diagnosis

The cardiac rhythm is atrial flutter (atrial rate: 260 beats per minute with varying A-V response (predominantly 2:1 A-V response), causing slightly irregular ventricular cycle. Ventricular tachycardia is simulated superficially because of broad QRS complexes as a result of RBBB. This patient had suffered from anteroseptal MI as well as diaphragmatic MI (Q waves are shown in leads V_1 and II) 6 months previously.

An artificial pacemaker is *not* indicated as long as there is no documented evidence of advanced bifascicular (BFB) or trifascicular block (TFB) (see Case 23), especially Mobitz type II A-V block or complete A-V block (even transient), and/or a history of near-syncope from bradyarrhythmia itself.

The patient was digitalized with rapid improvement.

Case 60

A 68-year-old woman was brought to the emergency room because of acute shortness of breath associated with marked weakness of a few hours duration. She denied chest pain and was not taking any medication.

1. *What is your ECG diagnosis?*
2. *What is the treatment of choice?*

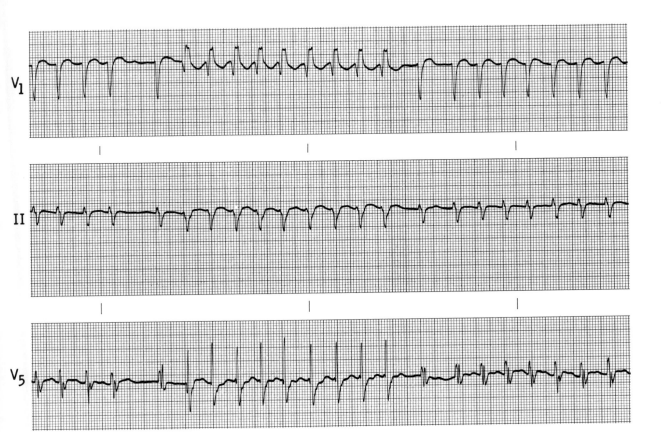

Case 60: Diagnosis

The cardiac rhythm is AF with rapid ventricular response (rate: 155–170 beats per minute). Note consecutively occurring bizarre QRS complexes due to AVC initiated by the Ashman's phenomenon (see Case 29). The R-R interval of the preceding cycle is very long just before the initiation of AVC—the characteristic feature of the Ashman's phenomenon (see Case 29).

A short run of ventricular tachycardia is closely simulated during consecutively occurring AVC, but a possibility of ventricular tachycardia is definitely excluded on the basis of 2 major findings—a lack of any ventricular pause following bizarre beats and the Ashman's phenomenon. Needless to say, it is extremely important to make a correct ECG rhythm diagnosis in order to provide an appropriate management.

The aberrantly conducted beats exhibit RBBB *pattern* with left anterior hemiblock (LAHB) *pattern* causing a BFB *pattern*. Of course, this ECG finding is *functional* BFB—*not* true or anatomic BFB.

She has improved markedly following rapid digitalization.

Case 61

This ECG tracing was obtained from a 51-year-old woman with chronic congestive heart failure. Her cardiologist has noticed that her cardiac rhythm had changed suddenly.

1. *What is your ECG diagnosis?*
2. *What is the most common cause of this arrhythmia?*

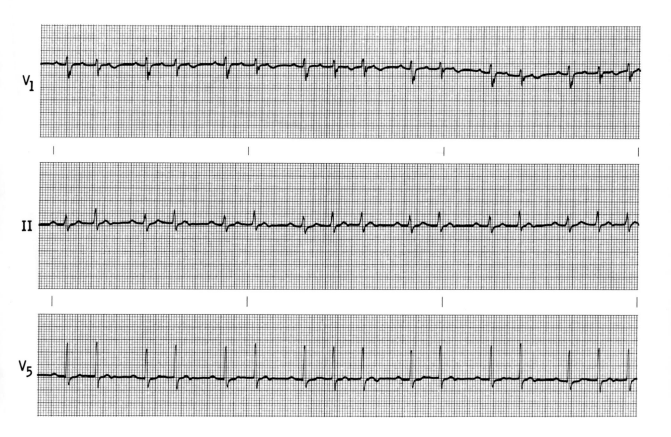

Case 61: Diagnosis

The cardiac rhythm is atrial tachycardia (atrial rate: 150 beats per minute) with varying (3:2 and 4:3) Wenckebach (Mobitz type I) A-V block causing a regular irregularity of the ventricular cycle (see Case 37). In addition, some QRS complexes are slightly bizarre because of AVC—Ashman's phenomenon (see Case 29). Atrial tachycardia with A-V block (most commonly Wenckebach A-V block) has been termed "PAT with block" by some cardiologists.

The etiologic factor for atrial tachycardia with Wenckebach A-V block is nearly always digitalis intoxication (see Chapter 7).

Discontinuation of digitalis will be the treatment of choice under this circumstance.

Case 62

Digitalis toxicity was suspected on a 39-year-old man with idiopathic cardiomyopathy.

What is your ECG diagnosis?

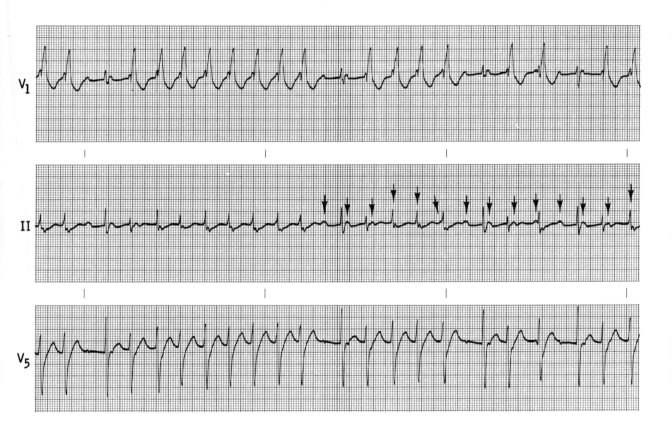

Case 62: Diagnosis

Arrows indicate ectopic P waves. The cardiac rhythm is atrial tachycardia (rate: 163 beats per minute) with slowly progressing Wenckebach A-V block of varying conduction ratio (see Case 37). It is obvious that many QRS complexes are bizarre and broad due to AVC initiated by the Ashman's phenomenon (see Case 29). Ventricular tachycardia is closely simulated during consecutively occurring AVC. As stressed previously, RBBB *pattern* is observed in 80–85% of all cases showing AVC (see Case 29).

The R wave in normally conducted beats is relatively tall, suggestive of right ventricular hypertrophy. In fact, this patient was found to have biventricular hypertrophy on chest X-ray films.

Case 63

A 78-year-old woman with hypertensive heart disease associated with chronic congestive heart failure has been taking digoxin 0.125 mg. and hydrochlorothiazide 25 mg. daily for several years.

What is your ECG diagnosis?

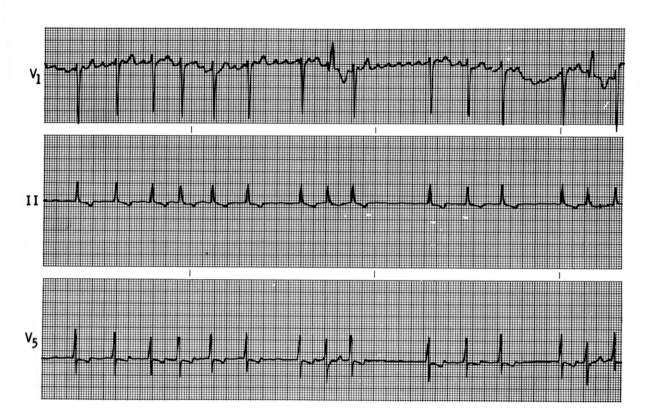

Case 63: Diagnosis

The cardiac rhythm shows atrial flutter-fibrillation with the ventricular rate ranging from 60 to 100 beats per minute. There are two bizarre QRS complexes with RBBB *pattern*. These bizarre QRS complexes are due to AVC as a result of Ashman's phenomenon (see Case 29).

The possibility of VPCs is absolutely excluded:

(a) because there is no ventricular pause following the bizarre beats and

(b) because of Ashman's phenomenon.

A 51-year-old man was admitted to the hospital because of rapid heart action.

What is your ECG diagnosis?

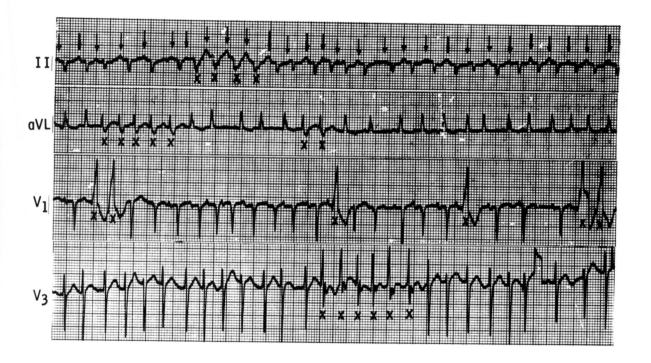

Case 64: Diagnosis

Arrows indicate P waves. This ECG tracing shows MAT with intermittent AVC (marked X). Ventricular premature beats and ventricular tachycardia are closely simulated when AVC occurs.

MAT is diagnosed because of varying P-P cycles with different P wave configurations. The diagnostic criteria of MAT have been described previously (see Case 54). AVC is confirmed by the following findings:

(a) No postectopic pause following bizarre QRS complex

(b) Varying ventricular cycles during bizarre QRS complexes

(c) RBBB pattern in bizarre QRS complexes

(d) Ashman's phenomenon

(e) P waves preceding bizarre QRS complexes

These findings are incompatible with ventricular premature beats or ventricular tachycardia. MAT is often refractory to various antiarrhythmic drugs, digitalis, and even DC shock. Thus, improvement of the underlying disease (commonly chronic lung disease) is much more effective in terminating this arrhythmia.

Case 65

A 44-year-old man with a history of MI 2 months earlier was seen in the emergency room because of an extremely rapid heart rate. He was not taking any drugs. He complained of weakness and dizziness, but his blood pressure was stable (130/85 mm. Hg.).

1. *What is the cardiac rhythm diagnosis?*
2. *What is the treatment of choice?*

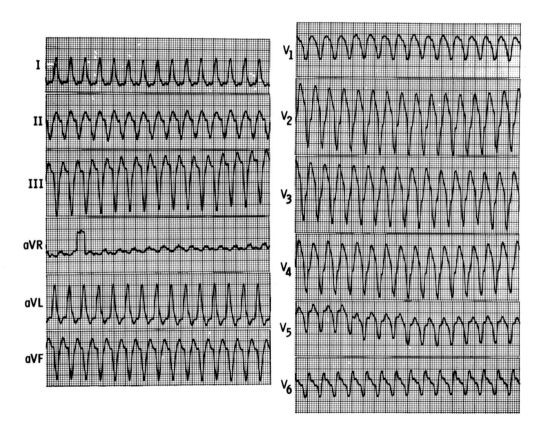

Case 65: Diagnosis

The cardiac rhythm is atrial flutter with a 1:1 A-V conduction (rate: 250 beats per minute) and an AVC which occurs because the ventricular rate is extremely rapid. The bizarre and broad QRS complexes mimic ventricular tachycardia. As a rule, ventricular tachycardia does not produce a rate over 200 beats per minute.

The treatment of choice is immediate DC shock. If DC shock is not available, rapid digitalization is then the treatment of choice. Alternatively, intravenous propranolol (Inderal) may be effective.

Case 66

A 23-year-old female was seen in the emergency room because of palpitations. She had suffered from similar episodes ever since her childhood, but she was not taking any medication regularly.

1. *What is the cardiac rhythm diagnosis?*
2. *What is the underlying disorder responsible for the production of this arrhythmia?*
3. *What is the treatment of choice?*

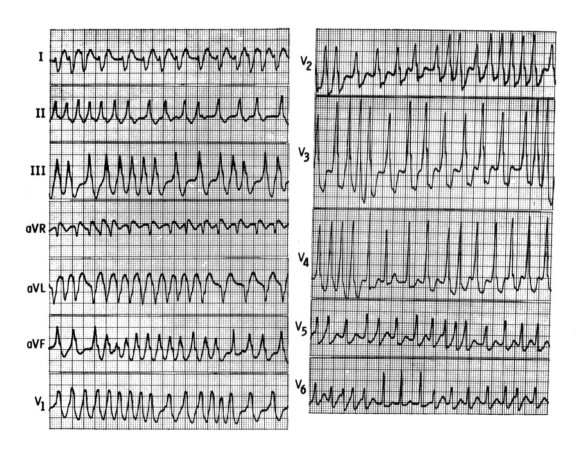

Case 66: Diagnosis

The cardiac rhythm is AF with very rapid ventricular response (ventricular rate: 200–300 beats per minute). The QRS complexes are extremely bizarre because almost all cardiac impulses are conducted to the ventricles via an anomalous pathway. The underlying disorder responsible for the production of this arrhythmia is, needless to say, Wolff-Parkinson-White (WPW) syndrome, type A. Detailed descriptions regarding the WPW syndrome are found elsewhere in this Book (see Chapter 6).

When the clinical situation is extremely urgent, immediate application of DC shock is the treatment of choice. Otherwise, intravenous injection of lidocaine (Xylocaine) will be the drug of choice (50–100 mg.). Even after termination of AF with anomalous A-V conduction, a long-term oral antiarrhythmic agent (e.g., quinidine, procainamide, or Norpace) is indicated for the prevention of the arrhythmia in most cases.

Propranolol (Inderal) is ineffective under this circumstance, and digitalis is contraindicated. It is extremely important to remember that the clinical situation often becomes worse when digitalis is given to the patient with AF with anomalous A-V conduction because digitalis enhances the conduction via an anomalous pathway leading to faster ventricular rate. In some cases, ventricular fibrillation may be provoked by digitalis under this circumstance.

AF with anomalous A-V conduction closely simulates ventricular tachycardia or even ventricular fibrillation.

Case 67

This ECG tracing was obtained from a 43-year-old man with several episodes of palpitations in the past few weeks. He was not taking any drug.

1. *What is the cardiac rhythm diagnosis?*
2. *What are the common underlying disorders responsible for the production of this arrhythmia?*

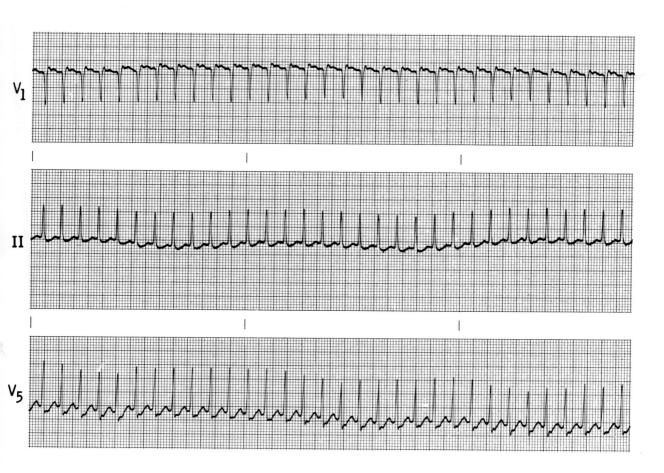

Case 67: Diagnosis

The cardiac rhythm is atrial flutter with 1:1 A-V conduction causing a very rapid ventricular rate (rate: 250 beats per minute). Note that the ventricular cycle is regular and the QRS complexes are normal (narrow). In general, atrial flutter waves are not readily visible when there is 1:1 A-V conduction. Under this circumstance, the atrial flutter cycle can be easily unmasked when the ventricular rate is slowed by carotid sinus stimulation or drugs (such as digitalis or propranolol).

Atrial flutter with 1:1 A-V conduction is extremely rare in adults although it is not uncommon in infants and young children. In adults, common underlying disorders to produce this arrhythmia may include hyperthyroidism, WPW syndrome, and any clinical situations with high catecholamine level. Atrial flutter with 1:1 A-V conduction occasionally occurs following a major cardiac surgery. This patient was found to have mild hyperthyroidism, and propranolol (Inderal) was effective to terminate the arrhythmia.

Case 68

These ECG rhythm strips were taken on a 43-year-old woman with known rheumatic heart disease. She was taking digoxin (0.25 mg. once daily) and an antiarrhythmic agent for her arrhythmia.

1. *What is your cardiac rhythm diagnosis?*
2. *What antiarrhythmic agent most likely is this patient taking?*

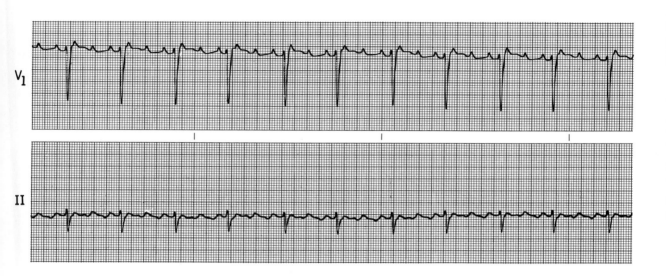

V₁

II

Case 68: Diagnosis

The cardiac rhythm is atrial flutter (atrial rate: 204 beats per minute) with 3:1 A-V block (ventricular rate: 68 beats per minute). The atrial flutter cycle is much slower than usual because of quinidine effect. Remember that the usual atrial flutter cycle ranges from 250 to 350 beats per minute (see Case 57).

Quinidine characteristically causes slowing of the atrial flutter cycle by virtue of the prolongation of the refractory period in the atria as a consequence of the drug's electrophysiologic property. Procainamide (Pronestyl) or Norpace (disopyramide) possesses a similar effect on the atria but its electrophysiologic action is less striking. Even though the atrial flutter cycle is much slower than usual due to quinidine effect in this ECG tracing, the characteristic flutter wave showing sawtooth appearance confirms the diagnosis of atrial flutter. In fact, the original flutter cycle before the administration of quinidine was 280 beats per minute in this patient.

By and large, a pure atrial flutter nearly always shows 2:1 A-V conduction (see Case 57), and the A-V conduction often becomes 4:1 when digitalis or propranolol (Inderal) is given (see Case 69). In addition, atrial flutter not uncommonly discloses Wenckebach A-V conduction or varying A-V conduction (see Cases 58 and 59). Atrial flutter with 3:1 or 5:1 A-V block is rather unusual mode of A-V conduction.

Case 69

This ECG tracing was obtained from a 79-year-old woman with chronic congestive heart failure due to hypertensive heart disease. She had been taking digoxin 0.125 mg. daily and hydrochlorothiazide 50 mg. every other day.

1. *What is the cardiac rhythm diagnosis?*
2. *What is the other ECG abnormality?*
3. *Is digitalis toxicity suspected?*

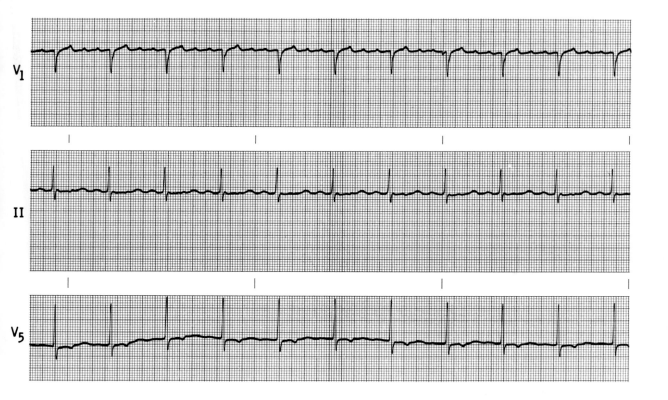

Case 69: Diagnosis

The cardiac rhythm is atrial flutter (atrial rate: 272 beats per minute) with 4:1 A-V block (ventricular rate: 68 beats per minute). Note a precisely regular ventricular cycle because every 4th flutter wave is conducted to the ventricle rhythmically throughout the tracing.

When digitalis is given to the patient with atrial flutter with 2:1 A-V conduction (see Case 57), the A-V conduction is often delayed so that 4:1 A-V block is the usual end result if atrial flutter persists. On the other hand, digitalis may terminate atrial flutter and may restore sinus rhythm. Otherwise, digitalis may transform atrial flutter to atrial fibrillation because the drug possesses an electrophysiologic property on the atria to shorten the atrial refractory period. This action of digitalis on the atria is exactly opposite to that of quinidine. Remember that atrial flutter cycle often slows down when quinidine is given (see Case 68).

Note a prominent U wave (clearly shown in lead II) indicative of hypokalemia (her serum potassium was found to be 3.2 mEq./L). In addition, there is nonspecific abnormality of S-T segment and T wave and/or digitalis effect.

Digitalis toxicity is extremely unlikely when dealing with 4:1 A-V block in atrial flutter. When A-V conduction is further delayed beyond 4:1 A-V block leading to more advanced A-V block, however, digitalis toxicity should be strongly considered (see Chapter 7). Her serum digoxin level was reported to be 1.0 ng./ml. (therapeutic range: 1.0–2.5 ng./ml.).

Case 70

This ECG tracing was recorded on a 78-year-old man with chronic congestive heart failure due to hypertensive heart disease. He was taking digoxin 0.125 mg. once and quinidine 0.3 g. 4 times daily.

What is the cardiac rhythm diagnosis?

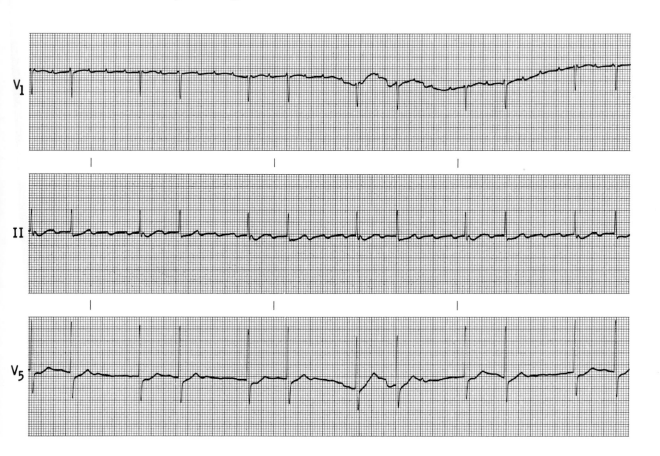

Case 70: Diagnosis

The cardiac rhythm is atrial flutter (atrial rate: 200 beats per minute) with Wenckebach A-V conduction (alternating 4:1 and 2:1 conduction). Note a regular irregularity of the ventricular cycle—alternating short and long R-R intervals. It should be noted that the long R-R interval is shorter than 2 short R-R intervals because the long R-R interval is shorter than 4 flutter cycles while the short R-R interval is longer than two flutter cycles. These ECG findings are the characteristic features of Wenckebach A-V conduction (see Case 37).

As described previously, slow atrial flutter cycle in this patient is due to quinidine effect (see Case 68). Remember that the usual atrial flutter cycle ranges from 250 to 350 beats per minute (see Case 57).

Case 71

This ECG tracing was taken at a general medical clinic for an annual medical check-up on a 72-year-old woman.

What is your cardiac rhythm diagnosis?

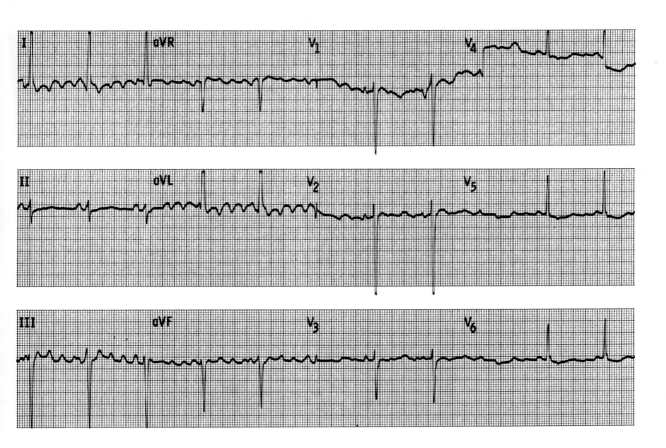

Case 71: Diagnosis

On superficial examination, the cardiac rhythm appears to be atrial flutter with 4:1 A-V block. However, it becomes obvious that the cardiac rhythm is actually normal sinus rhythm with a rate of 63 beats per minute by close observation. The pseudoatrial flutter waves are more pronounced in the extremity (limb) leads as a result of muscle tremors this patient has as a manifestation of Parkinson's disease. The sinus P waves are clearly shown in leads II and precordial leads.

In addition, left ventricular hypertrophy can be diagnosed without any difficulty.

Case 72

This ECG tracing was obtained from a 54-year-old man with chronic congestive heart failure due to hypertensive heart disease. He had been taking digoxin 0.25 mg. and hydrochlorothiazide 100 mg. daily for several months.

1. *What is your cardiac rhythm diagnosis?*
2. *What is most likely responsible for the production of this arrhythmia?*

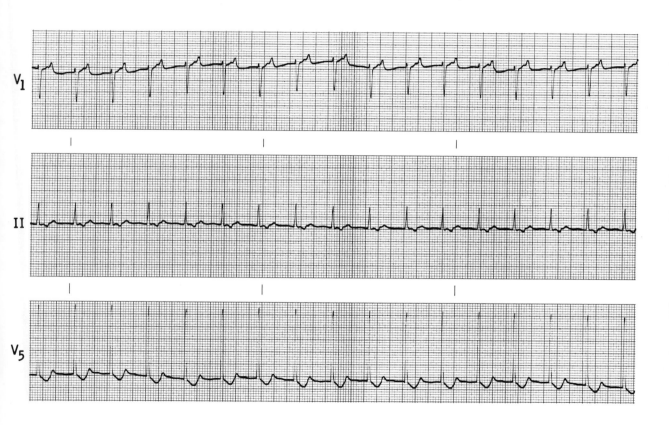

Case 72: Diagnosis

The cardiac rhythm diagnosis is nonparoxysmal A-V junctional tachycardia with a rate of 106 beats per minute. Note that each QRS complex is followed by a retrograde P wave and the cardiac cycle is precisely regular. Thus, an alternative cardiac rhythm diagnosis will be a reciprocating (re-entrant) tachycardia. It has been shown that almost all cases showing A-V junctional tachycardia are considered to be due to a re-entry mechanism in view of electrophysiologic study.

Two most common causes of nonparoxysmal A-V junctional tachycardia include digitalis intoxication and acute diaphragmatic MI (see Chapters 5 and 7). In this patient, digitalis toxicity is responsible for the production of nonparoxysmal A-V junctional tachycardia. His serum digoxin level was reported to be 3.4 ng./ml. (therapeutic range: 1.0–2.5 ng./ml.).

In addition, there is evidence of left ventricular hypertrophy.

Case 73

This ECG tracing was taken on a 20-year-old man with rheumatic aortic stenosis a few hours following surgical replacement of the aortic valve. He was not taking any medication except for a prophylactic penicillin therapy.

1. *What is your ECG diagnosis?*
2. *What is the treatment of choice?*

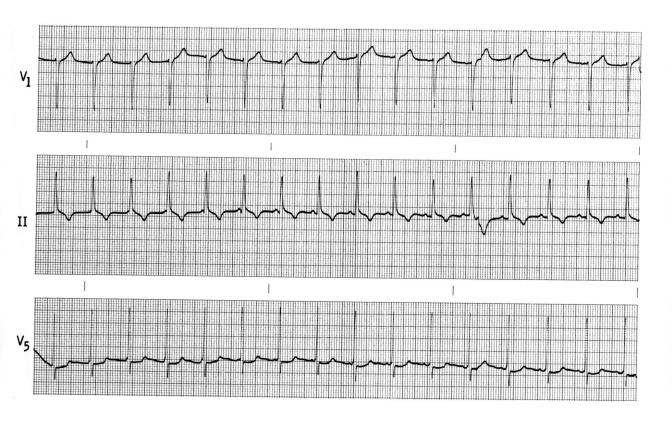

Case 73: Diagnosis

The cardiac rhythm is sinus with intermittent nonparoxysmal A-V junctional tachycardia, producing incomplete A-V dissociation. It is interesting to note that the atrial and ventricular rate are almost identical (rate: 96 beats) but independent at least in three-fourths of the tracing. The last few beats are most likely normally conducted sinus beats (ventricular captured beats). Therefore, the term "incomplete" A-V dissociation is used. In other words, *complete* A-V dissociation means that the atria and the ventricles beat independently throughout, whereas *incomplete* A-V dissociation means that there are occasional relationships between the atrial and ventricular activity and otherwise independent—meaning occasional occurrences of ventricular or atrial captured beats as seen in this tracing.

The term "isorhythmic A-V dissociation" is used by some cardiologists when the atrial and ventricular rates are very similar but independent. A-V dissociation, of course, means that there is no relationship between the atrial and ventricular activity. In this case, the underlying cause to produce A-V dissociation is an acceleration of the A-V junctional impulse formation—nonparoxysmal A-V junctional tachycardia.

As described previously (see Case 72), nonparoxysmal A-V junctional tachycardia is very common in patients with acute diaphragmatic MI (see Chapter 5) and digitalis intoxication (see Chapter 7). In addition, nonparoxysmal A-V junctional tachycardia is not uncommon within a few hours to a few days following any major cardiac surgery. No active treatment is required for postoperative nonparoxysmal A-V junctional tachycardia.

The diagnosis of left ventricular hypertrophy can be made without any difficulty on this tracing—a common finding in aortic stenosis.

Case 74

This ECG tracing was obtained from a 55-year-old woman with chronic obstructive pulmonary disease. She was not taking any drug.

1. *What is your cardiac rhythm diagnosis?*
2. *What is the treatment of choice?*

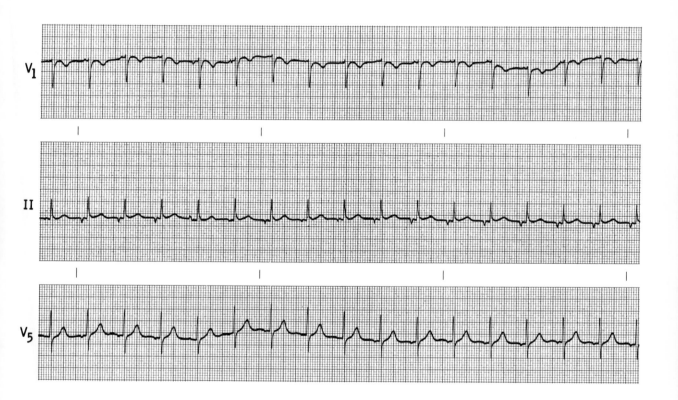

Case 74: Diagnosis

The cardiac rhythm is wandering atrial pacemaker between the sinus node and A-V junction (or left atrium) with a rate of 100 beats per minute. Note that the configuration of the P waves varies considerably (from upright to inverted P waves), but the P-R intervals and the P-P or (R-R) cycles remain relatively constant. This cardiac arrhythmia is considered to be a precursor of MAT. Common occurrence of MAT in patients with chronic obstructive pulmonary diseases has been emphasized previously (see Cases 54 and 64).

No treatment is indicated for wandering atrial pacemaker.

Case 75

Digitalis toxicity was suspected on 43-year-old man with rheumatic heart disease with mild congestive heart failure.

1. *What is your cardiac rhythm diagnosis?*
2. *What is the treatment of choice?*

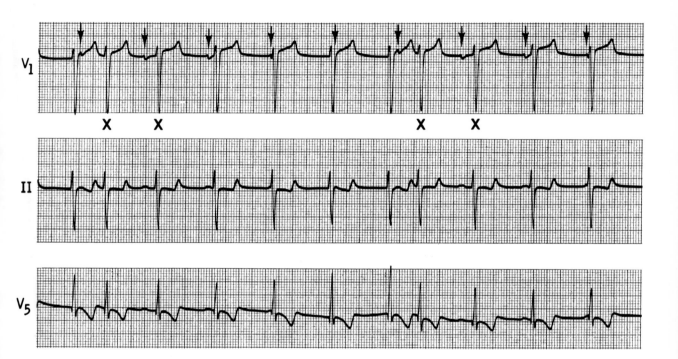

Case 75: Diagnosis

Arrows indicate sinus P waves. The cardiac rhythm is sinus (atrial rate: 64 beats per minute, indicated by arrows) with intermittent nonparoxysmal A-V junctional tachycardia (ventricular rate: 70 beats per minute) producing incomplete A-V dissociation. Note occasional ventricular captured beats (normally conducted sinus beats, marked X). Again, the underlying cause for the production of A-V dissociation is an acceleration of the impulse formation in the A-V junction—nonparoxysmal A-V junctional tachycardia. A-V dissociation has been described previously (see Case 73).

For digitalis-induced nonparoxysmal A-V junctional tachycardia, no active treatment is indicated in most cases, except for discontinuation of digitalis. If serum potassium is found to be low, potassium administration will be beneficial for any patient with digitalis toxicity. Remember that hypokalemia frequently predisposes to digitalis intoxication (see Chapter 7).

The configuration of the QRS complexes varies considerably, especially in lead V_5, but the finding is primarily due to respiratory variations. The diagnosis of left ventricular hypertrophy as well as left atrial enlargement can be entertained on this ECG tracing.

Case 76

These ECG rhythm strips were taken on a 70-year-old woman who has been taking quinidine 300 mg. 4 times daily for several months for palpitations due to VPCs.

1. *What is the cardiac rhythm diagnosis?*
2. *What is the treatment of choice?*

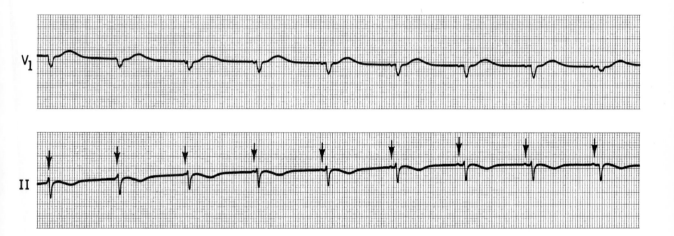

Case 76: Diagnosis

Arrows indicate the P waves of sinus origin. The cardiac rhythm is mild sinus bradycardia (atrial rate: 54 beats per minute, indicated by arrows) with independent A-V junctional escape rhythm (rate: 54 beats per minute) producing complete A-V dissociation. It is interesting to note that the rates of the atria and the ventricles are almost identical but independent throughout—meaning isorhythmic A-V dissociation.

The underlying mechanism responsible for the production of A-V dissociation in this case is the slowing of the sinus impulse formation—sinus bradycardia. A-V dissociation has been described in detail previously (see Case 73).

No treatment is indicated for her arrhythmia. Note the prolongation of the Q-T interval due to quinidine effect. Her VPCs subsided entirely after administration of quinidine.

Case 77

This ECG tracing was obtained from a 56-year-old man with coronary artery disease. He had suffered from a heart attack 3 months previously. He was not taking any drug.

1. *What is the cardiac rhythm diagnosis?*
2. *What is the origin of the ectopic beats?*
3. *What is the treatment of choice?*

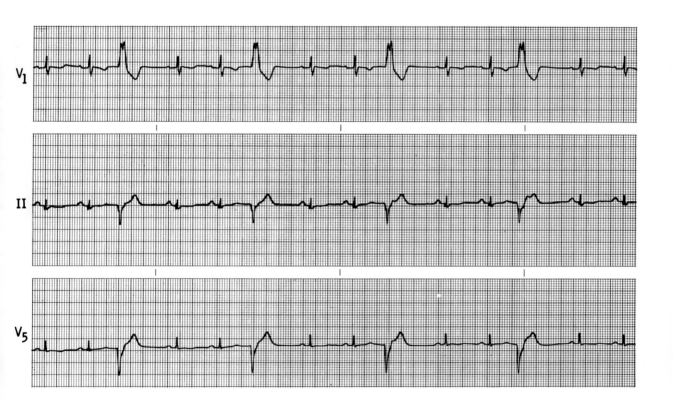

Case 77: Diagnosis

The underlying cardiac rhythm is sinus (rate: 82 beats per minute), but there are frequent VPCs producing ventricular trigeminy.

As far as the origin of the VPCs is concerned, it can be estimated with a reasonable certainty, judging from the morphology of the ectopic beats. In this ECG tracing, the VPCs are primarily upright (positive) in lead V_1 and downward (negative) in lead V_5, so that the configuration of the ectopic QRS complex resembles RBBB. By using a vectorial analysis, the VPCs are considered to be the left ventricular in origin because the ectopic impulse is moving toward the right precordial leads (e.g., lead V_1) and moving away from the left precordial leads (e.g., lead V_5).

It has been shown that the VPCs originating from the left ventricle as well as the ventricular septum (see Case 79) are much more common in elderly people and cardiac patients, particularly those with coronary artery disease and cardiomyopathy. On the other hand, right VPCs are much more common in young people and individuals without apparent heart disease (see Case 78). In digitalis intoxication, the VPCs are often multifocal, or originating from the left ventricle or the ventricular septum (see Chapter 7).

There is a general agreement that frequent VPCs should be treated when found in cardiac patients. Propranolol (Inderal) or quinidine should be tried first. If these agents are ineffective or contraindicated, procainamide (Pronestyl) or disopyramide (Norpace) may be tried.

Case 78

This ECG tracing was obtained from a 28-year-old healthy male as a part of an annual medical check-up. He was not complaining of any symptom and denied any unusual habit (e.g., excessive consumption of coffee, or alcohol, smoking, etc.).

1. *What is your cardiac rhythm diagnosis?*
2. *What is the origin of the ectopic beats?*
3. *What is the best approach to this cardiac arrhythmia?*

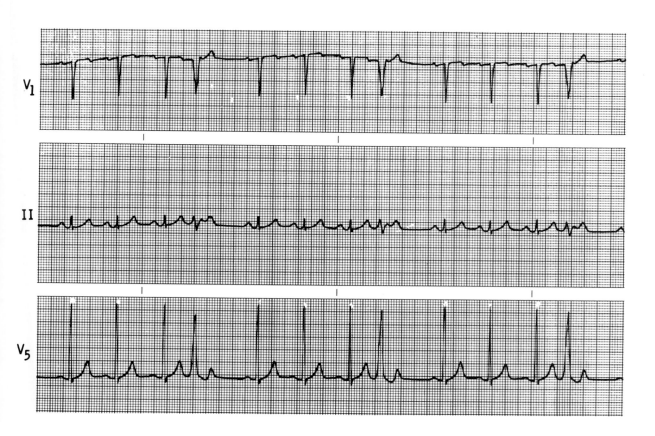

Case 78: Diagnosis

The underlying cardiac rhythm is sinus (rate: 85 beats per minute) but there are frequent VPCs producing ventricular quadrigeminy.

The VPCs in this tracing are considered to be the right ventricular in origin because the ectopic QRS complexes are downward (negative) in lead V_1 and upright (positive) in lead V_5. In order to satisfy these QRS configurations of the VPCs, the ectopic impulses must be moving away from the right precordium and moving toward the left precordium.

A relatively benign nature of the right VPCs has been described previously (see Case 77), but any possible etiologic factor should be investigated. Routine questions under this circumstance should include any unusual personal habit (e.g., excessive usage of coffee, tea, cola drinks, or alcohol, and cigarette smoking), emotional tension and possible underlying cardiac or noncardiac disorder. MVPS and hyperthyroidism should always be considered as a possible underlying disorder until proven otherwise.

By and large, active treatment is not considered to be indicated for asymptomatic healthy individuals with VPCs, even when they occur very frequently (30 VPCs or more per hour).

Case 79

This ECG tracing was taken on a 68-year-old woman because of palpitations with unpleasant feeling in the chest for a few weeks. She was not taking any drug and denied any other cardiac symptom.

1. *What is your cardiac rhythm diagnosis?*
2. *What is the origin of the ectopic beats?*
3. *What is the best therapeutic approach?*

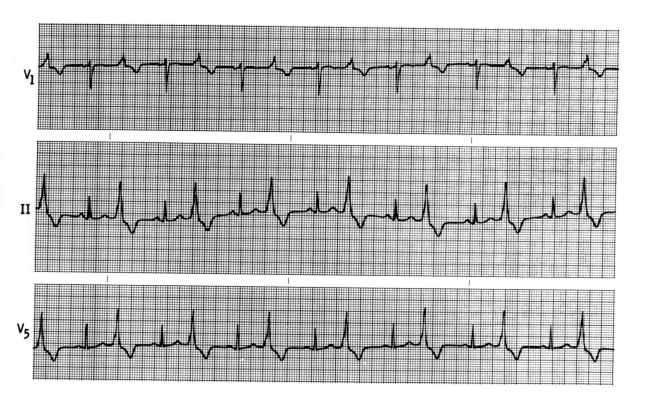

Case 79: Diagnosis

The underlying cardiac rhythm is sinus (rate: 94 beats per minute) but there are frequent VPCs producing ventricular bigeminy.

The VPCs in this case are considered to be originating from the ventricular septum judging from the configuration of the QRS complexes of the ectopic beats—upright (positive) in both left and right precordial leads.

As described previously (see Case 77), the clinical significance of the septal VPCs is the same as that of the left VPCs. Namely, the septal VPCs are common in elderly individuals, cardiac patients and digitalis intoxication.

When VPCs are symptomatic, regardless of the presence or absence of the underlying heart disease, one or more antiarrhythmic agents (e.g., propranolol, quinidine, etc.) should be administered. Investigation of possible underlying etiologic cause to produce VPCs should always be a part of medical management. When VPCs occur suddenly, a possibility of any acute cardiac event, particularly acute MI, must be raised, especially in older individuals or known cardiac patients.

Case 80

These ECG rhythm strips were taken on a 37-year-old man without apparent heart disease. He was not taking any medication.

1. *What is your ECG cardiac rhythm diagnosis?*
2. *What is the clinical significance of this arrhythmia?*

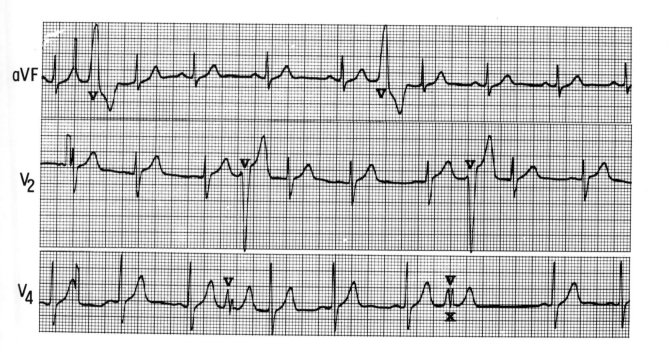

Case 80: Diagnosis

The underlying rhythm is sinus arrhythmia (rate: 69–80 beats per minute), but there are frequent VPCs (marked V). It is interesting to note that all VPCs are interpolated except one (marked X). The origin of the VPCs is considered to be the right ventricle, judging from predominantly negative (downward) QRS complexes in lead V_2 and positive (upright) QRS complexes in lead V_4.

The R-R interval which contains a VPC is longer than the basic R-R intervals because P-R interval of the sinus beat immediately following a VPC is prolonged as a result of a concealed retrograde ventriculoatrial conduction by a VPC. Namely, the A-V conduction system is partially refractory when the sinus inpulse is conducted soon after a VPC as a result of deep penetration of the ectopic impulse into the A-V junction, conducted in a retrograde fashion from the ventricular ectopic focus—called "retrograde ventriculoatrial concealed conduction."

Clinically, interpolated VPCs are considered to be benign; likewise right VPCs are benign clinically in most cases (see Case 78).

Case 81

This ECG tracing was obtained from a 69-year-old man with coronary and hypertensive heart disease. He had been taking digoxin 0.25 mg. and hydrochlorothiazide 50 mg. daily for chronic mild heart failure. Digitalis toxicity was suspected.

1. *What is your cardiac rhythm diagnosis?*
2. *What is the treatment of choice?*

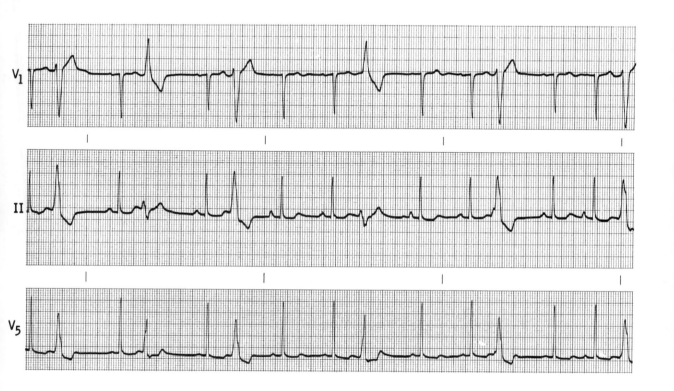

Case 81: Diagnosis

The underlying cardiac rhythm is sinus (rate: 72 beats per minute), but there are frequent multifocal VPCs as well as frequent APCs. It is interesting to note that a VPC and an APC occur on consecutive beats in some areas (e.g., the 3rd VPC followed by an APC). The recognition of APCs is relatively easy because they appear prematurely and the ectopic P wave is peaked and tall (different from sinus P wave).

Almost every known type of cardiac arrhythmias may be induced by digitalis toxicity, but multifocal VPCs are of the most common digitalis-induced arrhythmias (see Chapter 7). Needless to say, immediate discontinuation of digitalis is the treatment of choice when dealing with any patient with digitalis intoxication. When serum potassium is found to be low—a common occurrence during diuretic therapy in patients with digitalis toxicity—supplementary potassium administration is indicated. If VPCs persist, Dilantin (diphenylhydantoin) should be tried (see Chapter 7).

Case 82

These Holter monitor ECG rhythm strips were obtained from a 39-year-old hypertensive man who had suffered a diaphragmatic (inferior) MI 6 months earlier. The Holter monitor ECG was ordered because of palpitations. He was not taking any drugs. His 12-lead ECG reveals sinus rhythm, evidence of an old diaphragmatic MI and left ventricular hypertrophy (not shown here). No arrhythmia is observed on the 12-lead ECG.

1. *What is the cardiac rhythm diagnosis?*
2. *What is the treatment of choice?*

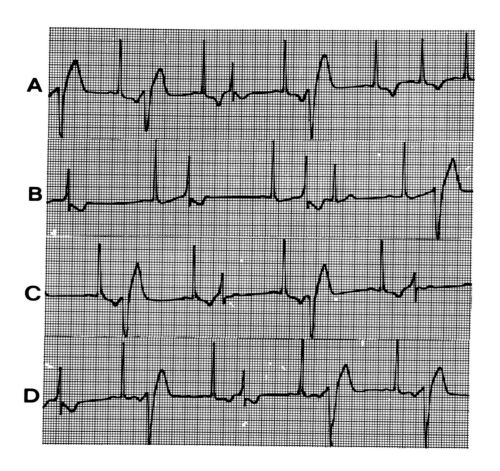

Case 82: Diagnosis

The rhythm strips A through D are not continuous. The Holter monitor ECG revealed sinus rhythm (rate: 85 beats per minute) and frequent multifocal VPCs with areas of ventricular bigeminy and ventricular group beats. Note that there are three or four different forms of VPCs.

It has been shown that multifocal VPCs are usually found in organic heart disease, particularly coronary heart disease and cardiomyopathy, and digitalis intoxication. Thus, multifocal VPCs are considered malignant, and they must be treated. The commonly used oral drugs include quinidine, and procainamide (Pronestyl) when these arrhythmias are associated with coronary heart disease or other forms of organic heart disease. Diphenylhydantoin (Dilantin), however, is the drug of choice for digitalis-induced ventricular arrhythmias.

Case 83

This ECG tracing was taken on a 57-year-old man with recent anterior MI. He developed a very rapid heart action (shown on the upper 2 strips) associated with hypotension. The lower strips were recorded following the termination of the tachyarrhythmia.

1. *What is your cardiac rhythm diagnosis?*
2. *What is the treatment of choice?*

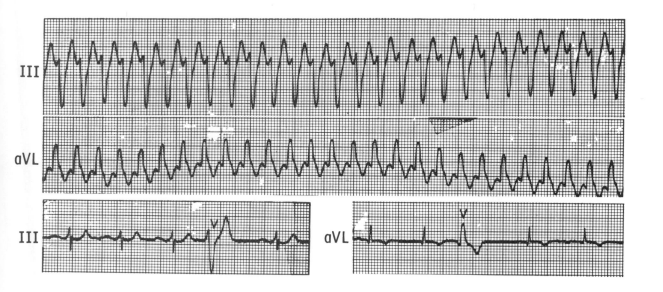

Case 83: Diagnosis

The cardiac rhythm diagnosis is paroxysmal ventricular tachycardia with a rate of 200 beats per minute. There is no discernible P wave during the tachycardia and the ventricular cycle is precisely regular. It is important to recognize that the QRS configuration in an isolated VPC (marked V) during sinus rhythm (lower strips) is identical to that during the tachycardia. This finding confirms that the tachycardia is unquestionably ventricular in origin—ventricular tachycardia.

The treatment of choice for ventricular tachycardia is immediate application of DC shock when there is a significant hemodynamic abnormality due to the tachycardia. Otherwise, intravenous injection of lidocaine (Xylocaine, 50–100 mg.) will be the treatment of choice. After the termination of ventricular tachycardia, a continuous intravenous infusion (1–5 mg per minute) of lidocaine is recommended for 24–48 hours to several days, depending upon the clinical circumstance.

Case 84

This ECG tracing was taken on a 59-year-old man with acute anterior MI. He developed this rapid heart action soon after admission to the coronary care unit.

1. *What is your cardiac rhythm diagnosis?*
2. *What is the exact origin of the ectopic impulse formation?*

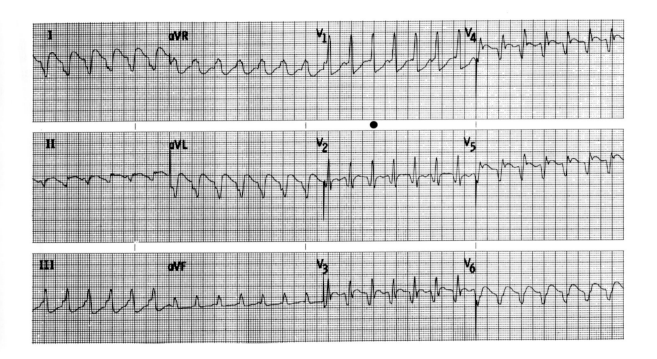

Case 84: Diagnosis

The cardiac rhythm diagnosis is paroxysmal ventricular tachycardia with a rate of 165 beats per minute. The ventricular cycle is precisely regular and there is no discernible P wave.

The determination of the site of the ventricular tachycardia can be made with the same way to determine the origin of a VPC. Namely, the analysis of the configuration of the QRS complexes during ventricular tachycardia from a vectorial approach enable the readers to determine the origin of the ectopic impulse formation (see Case 77). The ventricular tachycardia in this patient is considered to be the left ventricular in origin, judging from the upright (positive) QRS complexes in the right precordial leads and downward (negative) QRS complexes in the left precordial leads (see Case 77).

It has been shown that ventricular tachycardia of the left ventricular origin as well as the ventricular septal origin is much more common in patients with coronary artery disease, particularly in acute MI. In contrast, right ventricular tachycardia (see Case 85), if it occurs, is predominantly encountered in young individuals with no apparent heart disease. Of course, ventricular tachycardia originating from any site in the ventricles can occur in patients with a variety of heart disease. The treatment of paroxysmal ventricular tachycardia has been described previously (see Case 83).

Case 85

This ECG tracing was obtained from a 43-year-old apparently healthy man with no demonstrable heart disease. He was seen in the emergency room because of palpitations, but there was no other significant symptom or hemodynamic abnormality.

1. *What is your ECG diagnosis?*
2. *What is the origin of the ectopic impulse formation?*

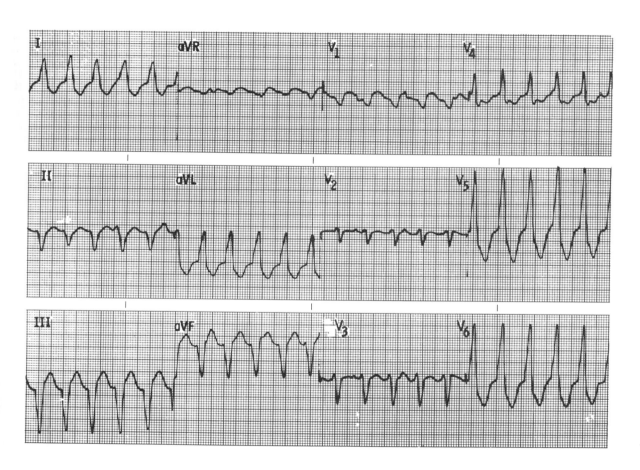

Case 85: Diagnosis

The cardiac rhythm is nonparoxysmal ventricular tachycardia (accelerated idioventricular rhythm or idioventricular tachycardia—meaning a relatively slow ventricular tachycardia) with a rate of 136 beats per minute. The P waves of the sinus origin can be identified by a careful analysis of the atrial mechanisms (see leads V_{1-3}). Thus, the complete diagnosis of this ECG tracing is sinus rhythm (atrial rate: 75 beats per minute) with independent nonparoxysmal ventricular tachycardia (ventricular rate: 136 beats per minute) producing complete A-V dissociation.

As far as the origin of this ventricular tachycardia is concerned, the same vectorial approach is applied as described earlier (see Cases 77, 78, and 84). That is, the tachycardia is considered to be arising from the right ventricle because the QRS complexes are predominantly downward (negative) in the right precordial leads and upright (positive) in the left precordial leads.

Relatively slow ventricular tachycardia (rate ranging from 70 to 150 beats per minute), which has been commonly termed "nonparoxysmal ventricular tachycardia" or "accelerated idioventricular rhythm," may be encountered in apparently healthy individuals. In most cases, nonparoxysmal ventricular tachycardia is self-limited, and it does not cause hemodynamic abnormality. When the individual is symptomatic (usually palpitations or strange sensation in the chest) from this slow ventricular tachycardia, however, one or more antiarrhythmic agents (e.g., propranolol, quinidine, or procainamide) should be tried. As a rule, any possible underlying cause for the development of the arrhythmia should always be investigated.

Case 86

This ECG tracing was obtained from a 54-year-old man with acute extensive anterior MI. He was relatively asymptomatic (other than the usual chest pain from acute MI) while he developed this arrhythmia.

1. *What is your cardiac rhythm diagnosis?*
2. *What is the origin of this arrhythmia?*
3. *What is the mechanism of this arrhythmia?*
4. *What is the treatment of choice?*

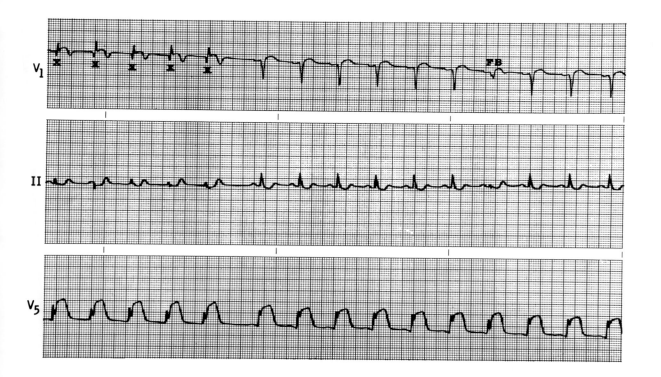

Case 86: Diagnosis

The underlying cardiac rhythm is sinus with a rate of 86 beats per minute. It is interesting to note that there are consecutively occurring bizarre QRS complexes with relatively narrow QRS configuration which shows incomplete RBBB *pattern* (marked X).

These bizarre QRS complexes are considered to be originating from one of the fascicles of the left bundle branch system. Note a ventricular fusion beat (marked FB). As far as the mechanism of this arrhythmia is concerned, it is most likely a parasystolic mechanism, in view of constant shortest interectopic intervals—meaning independent ectopic rhythm to the basic sinus rhythm. Therefore, a complete diagnosis of this arrhythmia is a parasystolic fascicular tachycardia with a rate of 88 beats per minute (rate is very similar to the sinus rate). The fascicular tachycardia is considered to be a form of ventricular tachycardia.

It has been shown that the fascicular tachycardia or parasystolic ventricular tachycardia is not uncommon in the first few days of acute MI. This relatively slow ventricular tachycardia is usually self-limited, and it disappears spontaneously in most cases. Accordingly, no treatment is necessary.

Case 87

These ECG rhythm strips were taken on a 38-year-old hypertensive man as a part of a routine follow-up check-up. He has been taking propranolol (Inderal) 30 mg. 4 times daily for his mild hypertension. He was asymptomatic while this ECG tracing was recorded.

1. *What is your cardiac rhythm diagnosis?*
2. *What is the treatment of choice?*
3. *What underlying disease process may be responsible for producing this arrhythmia?*

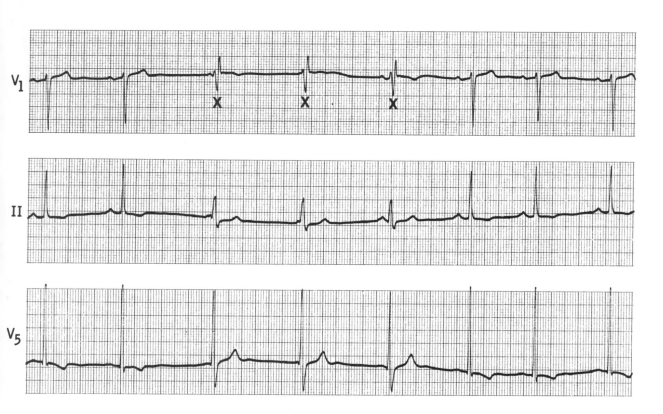

Case 87: Diagnosis

The underlying cardiac rhythm is sinus arrhythmia and sinus bradycardia (rate: 45–54 beats per minute) with slight first degree A-V block. There are three bizarre QRS complexes (marked X) independent to the basic sinus P waves so that incomplete A-V dissociation is produced. These bizarre QRS complexes represent ventricular escape beats (marked X) which may be arising from one of the fascicles of the left bundle branch system, judging from a relatively narrow QRS configuration which shows RBBB *pattern*.

No treatment is necessary for this arrhythmia because the ventricular escape beats occur as a result of sinus bradycardia secondary to propranolol therapy. However, a failure of the expected A-V junctional escape beats to appear during sinus bradycardia is a rather unusual phenomenon. Under this circumstance, diseased A-V node should be considered, although the dysfunctioning A-V node itself may also be due to propranolol therapy, at least in part. At any rate, further investigation is necessary for possible underlying diseased A-V node after discontinuation of propranolol. Remember that the diseased A-V node often coexists with dysfunctioning sinus node. Thus, a possibility of sick sinus syndrome should be strongly considered under this circumstance (see Chapter 1).

The diagnosis of left ventricular hypertrophy and left atrial enlargement can be made without any difficulty.

Case 88

A Holter monitor ECG was obtained from a 56-year-old woman with exertional chest pain associated with lightheadedness. She was hypertensive and had been taking hydrochlorothiazide (50 mg. daily). Her 12-lead ECG revealed a sinus rhythm and a nonspecific abnormality of the S-T, T wave changes (not shown here).

1. *What is the ECG diagnosis?*
2. *What is the treatment of choice?*

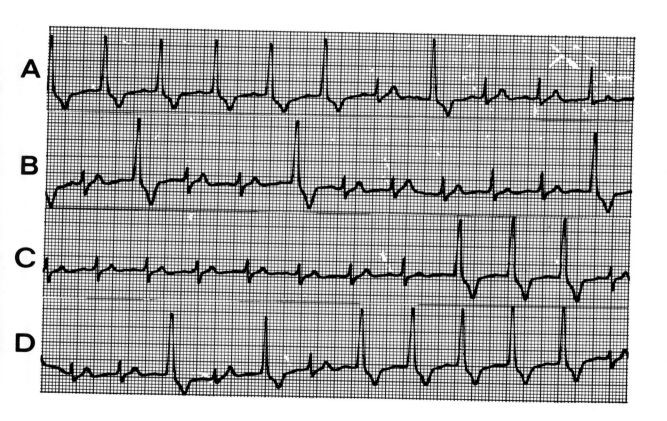

Case 88: Diagnosis

The rhythm strips A through D are not continuous. The cardiac rhythm is sinus arrhythmia with areas of sinus tachycardia (rate: 103–110 beats per minute). It is noteworthy that there are two types of QRS complexes due to an intermittent LBBB. Intermittent LBBB in this patient, however, was not related to the heart rate, since it was rate-independent.

Nonparoxysmal ventricular tachycardia (accelerated ventricular rhythm) is closely simulated during LBBB. The LBBB in this patient is, of course, an incidental finding and unrelated to her symptoms. Needless to say, no treatment is indicated.

Case 89

This ECG tracing was recorded on an 81-year-old man as a part of an annual medical check-up. He has been healthy for his age, but his ECG tracing shows several bizarre beats.

1. *What is your ECG diagnosis?*
2. *What is the treatment of choice?*

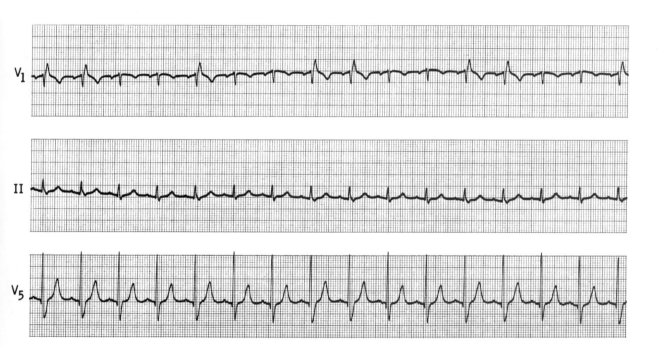

Case 89: Diagnosis

The cardiac rhythm is sinus with a rate of 94 beats per minute. There are bizarre QRS complexes which occur intermittently, unrelated to the basic heart rate. This finding obviously represents intermittent RBBB, which is rate-independent. Intermittent RBBB superficially resembles frequent VPCs with ventricular group beats.

Needless to say, no treatment is required for intermittent RBBB.

Case 90

A 58-year-old woman was brought to the emergency room because she suddenly developed a rapid heart action. Other than palpitations, she was relatively asymptomatic when she was examined in the emergency room, and her blood pressure was normal (135/90 mm. Hg.) She was not taking any drug.

An ECG tracing shown in this page (tracing A) was taken in the emergency room, whereas another ECG tracing shown in the next page (tracing B) was obtained following the termination of the tachycardia.

1. *What is the cardiac rhythm diagnosis during the rapid heart action?*
2. *What other ECG abnormality is present?*
3. *What is the proper therapeutic approach?*

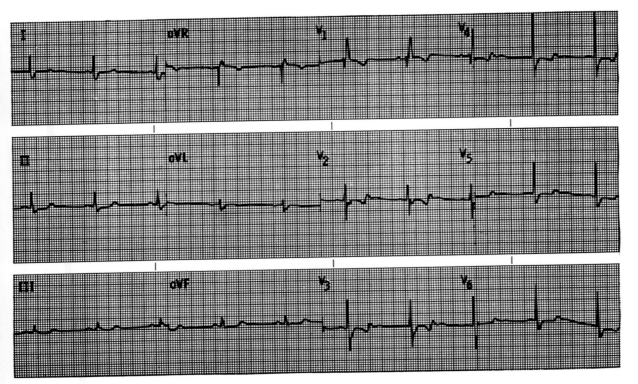

Case 90: Diagnosis

Tracing A: The cardiac rhythm is regular with a rate of 165 beats per minute, and the QRS complexes exhibit RBBB *pattern*. No P wave is discernible. Therefore, this tachycardia may be a supraventricular (either atrial or A-V junctional) tachycardia with RBBB, or ventricular tachycardia which may arise from one of the fascicles of the left bundle branch system, judging from the QRS morphology showing RBBB *pattern*. However, supraventricular tachycardia with the pre-existing RBBB is confirmed, because another ECG tracing taken during sinus rhythm (tracing B) shows an identical QRS configuration as the tachycardia QRS morphology—the pre-existing RBBB.

Tracing B: Sinus bradycardia (rate: 54 beats per minute) with RBBB.

Treatment: When dealing with any unknown regular tachycardia, the first therapeutic approach is carotid sinus stimulation (CSS), providing that the patient is not taking digitalis. CSS is often effective for terminating paroxysmal supraventricular (atrial or A-V junctional) tachycardia. When the arrhythmia is ventricular tachycardia, there is no response to CSS. It should be noted that CSS may not be effective for supraventricular tachycardia in some cases. Thus, no-response to CSS does not favor or exclude the diagnosis of supraventricular or ventricular tachycardia.

When the clinical situation is urgent, immediate application of DC shock will be the treatment of choice. After the termination of various tachyarrhythmias, many patients may require one or more antiarrhythmic agents (e.g., quinidine, propranolol, procainamide, etc.) to prevent the recurrence of the arrhythmia.

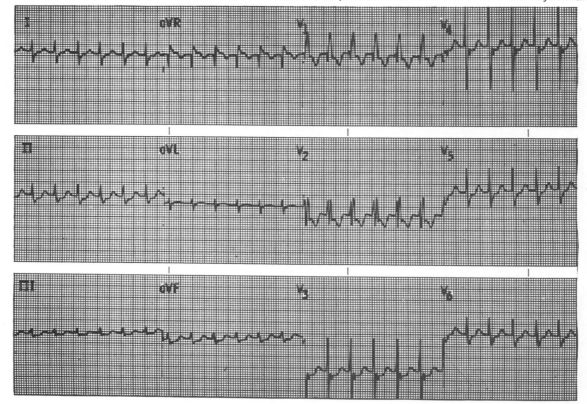

These ECG rhythm strips were obtained from a 74-year-old woman with several fainting episodes. She was not taking any medication.

1. *What is your cardiac rhythm diagnosis?*
2. *What is the treatment of choice?*

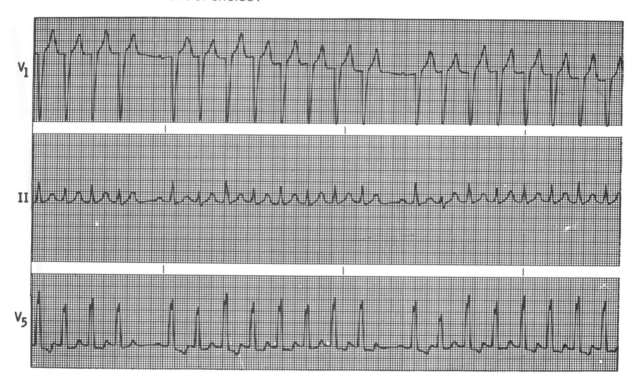

Case 91: Diagnosis

The underlying cardiac rhythm is sinus tachycardia (atrial rate: 128 beats per minute), but there are periodic ventricular pauses. This ECG finding represents Mobitz type II A-V block. The QRS complexes are broad because of LBBB. Note that the P-R intervals of all conducted beats are constant until blocked P waves occur—the characteristic feature of Mobitz type II A-V block (see Chapter 3).

An interesting ECG finding in this tracing is occurrence of bizarre QRS complex following each ventricular pause. This finding represents AVC due to the Ashman's phenomenon (see Case 29). Namely, the aberrantly conducted QRS complex is different from the remaining QRS complexes because the pre-existing LBBB is altered again as a result of the Ashman's phenomenon.

The treatment of choice is, of course, permanent artificial pacemaker implantation because Mobitz type II A-V block represents infranodal block [incomplete bilateral bundle branch block (BBBB) or incomplete TFB—see Case 23] which is irreversible.

Case 92

A 73-year-old woman was seen at the neurologic clinic for a routine check-up. The ECG tracing shown in this page (tracing A) was taken before treatment, whereas another ECG tracing, shown in the next page (tracing B), was recorded after treatment.

1. *What is your ECG diagnosis in both tracings?*
2. *What is most likely the underlying disorder responsible for the production of this ECG finding?*

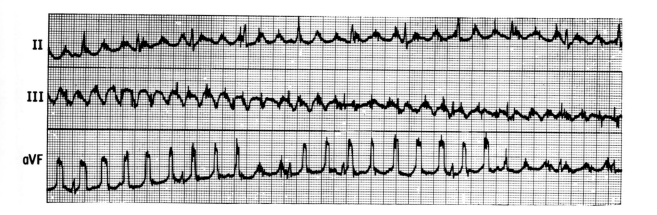

Case 92: Diagnosis

Tracing A: On superficial examination, the cardiac rhythm appears to be atrial flutter or even ventricular tachycardia in some areas. However, this ECG finding is produced by artifacts—muscle tremors of the extremities. It is possible to recognize the underlying sinus rhythm by a careful examination.

This woman has been suffering from Parkinson's disease, which was responsible for the production of this ECG finding. After treatment, normal sinus rhythm is recorded without any muscle tremors (see tracing B).

Tracing B: Normal sinus rhythm with a rate of 74 beats per minute, and the artifacts due to muscle tremors are no longer present after treatment.

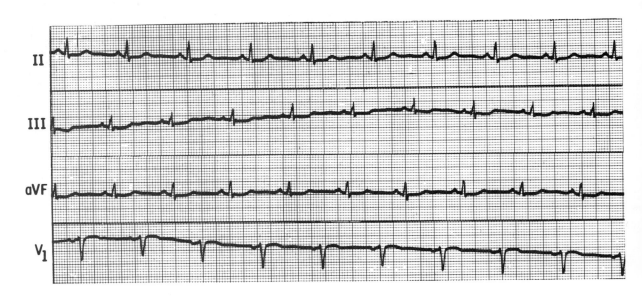

Case 93

These ECG rhythm strips were recorded via a cardiac monitor in the coronary care unit. Leads II-a and b are continuous.

What is your ECG diagnosis?

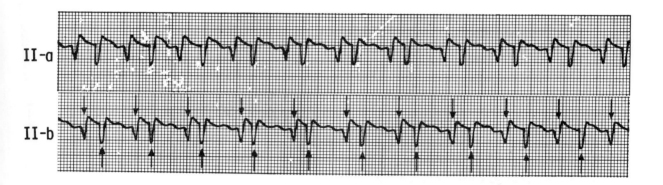

Case 93: Diagnosis

On superficial examination the cardiac rhythm appears to be a complex cardiac arrhythmia (e.g., frequent VPCs, ventricular parasystole, etc.). In reality, the electrical activities of 2 patients are recorded simultaneously (indicated by upward and downward arrows) via a cardiac monitor.

When dealing with any cardiac arrhythmia, a possibility of various artifacts must always be considered, especially when the mechanism of a given arrhythmia is difficult to ascertain. Needless to say, an erroneous diagnosis of a given cardiac arrhythmia frequently leads to improper treatment.

chapter 5

Cardiac Arrhythmias Associated with Myocardial Infarction

Case 94

A 56-year-old man with a previous heart attack was admitted to the coronary care unit because of chest pain several hours in duration. He was not taking any drug except for aspirin, 2 tablets daily. He was not complaining of dizziness, near-syncope, or syncope, and his blood pressure was stable (130/85 mm. Hg.).

The ECG tracing shown in this page (tracing A) was taken on admission, whereas another ECG tracing, shown on the next page (tracing B), was recorded 12 hours later.

1. What is your diagnosis of both ECG tracings?
2. Is his cardiac arrhythmia due to anterior myocardial infarction (MI) or diaphragmatic MI?
3. Is an artificial pacemaker indicated?

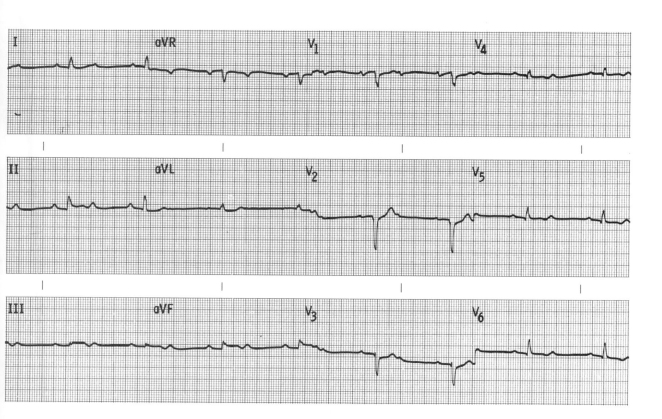

Case 94: Diagnosis

Tracing A: The cardiac rhythm is sinus (atrial rate: 96 beats per minute) with 2:1 A-V block (ventricular rate: 48 beats per minute). When dealing with 2:1 A-V block with normal QRS complexes, the block is a variant of Wenckebach (Mobitz type I) A-V block (see Cases 37 and 95). Thus, the A-V block represents A-V nodal block (a block in the A-V node itself) under this circumstance. As repeatedly stressed, Wenckebach A-V block is common in acute diaphragmatic MI because the blood supply to the A-V junction is often impaired, leading to a transient ischemia in the A-V junction (see Case 95). Wenckebach A-V block (or 2:1 A-V block as a variant of Wenckebach A-V block) in acute diaphragmatic MI is usually self-limited, and the A-V block disappears within few hours or days spontaneously. In fact, his A-V conduction improved progressively, and Wenckebach A-V block has changed to first degree A-V block within 12 hours spontaneously (see tracing B).

This patient had suffered from anterior MI 6 months previously, and recent diaphragmatic MI was responsible for the production of 2:1 A-V block (a variant of Wenckebach A-V block).

Tracing B: The ECG tracing taken 12 hours later discloses sinus rhythm (rate: 95 beats per minute) with first degree A-V block (P-R interval: 0.24 second).

The diagnosis of old extensive anterior MI and recent diaphragmatic MI can be made without any

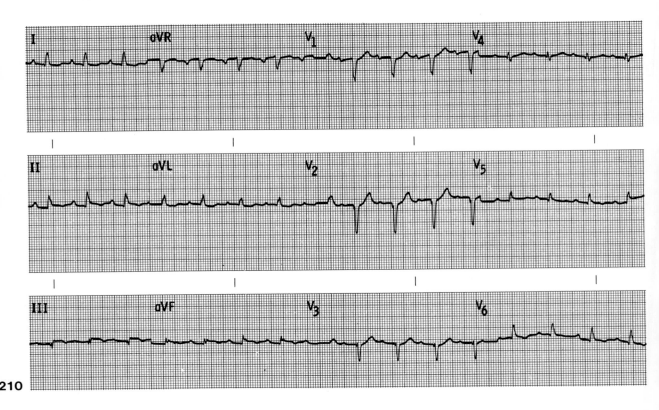

difficulty. In addition, a low voltage of the QRS complexes is readily recognized. The term "low voltage" is used when a sum of the QRS complexes (both upright and negative components) in standard leads (leads I, II, and III) is 15 mm. or less. Low voltage is very common in patients with MI.

Treatment: In most cases, artificial pacemaker is *not* indicated for 2:1 A-V block (a variant of Wenckebach A-V block) due to diaphragmatic MI because the A-V block is usually transient and self-limited. A temporary artificial pacing may be indicated only rarely when the ventricular rate is so slow (the rate slower than 40 and often less than 35 beats per minute) that the patient develops significant symptoms (e.g., dizziness, near-syncope, or syncope) and/or hemodynamic abnormalities (e.g., hypotension).

These cardiac rhythm strips shown were recorded from a 62-year-old man in the coronary care unit. Leads II-a and b are continuous.

1. *What is your cardiac rhythm diagnosis?*
2. *What is the underlying heart disease?*
3. *What is the treatment of choice?*

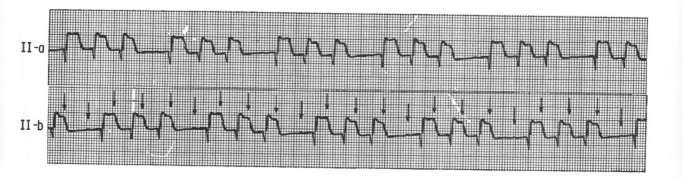

Case 95: Diagnosis

The arrows indicate sinus P waves. The cardiac rhythm is marked sinus tachycardia (atrial rate: 146 beats per minute) with 4:3 Wenckebach (Mobitz type I) A-V block. Many P waves are superimposed on the S-T segment and T waves, falsely suggesting absent P waves. Three ventricular grouped beats are followed by a ventricular pause, and this cardiac cycle repeats itself throughout the tracing. The mechanism of Wenckebach A-V block has been fully described previously (see Case 37).

Note the marked S-T segment elevation with pathologic Q waves diagnostic of acute diaphragmatic MI. As emphasized previously, transient Wenckebach A-V block is common during early phase of acute diaphragmatic MI. No hemodynamic alteration is produced, so that in most cases no treatment is indicated for the Wenckebach A-V block associated with acute diaphragmatic MI.

Case 96

A 76-year-old woman was admitted to the coronary care unit because of recent diaphragmatic MI. She was not taking any medication.

1. *What is your cardiac rhythm diagnosis?*
2. *What is the mechanism for altering the underlying cardiac arrhythmia?*
3. *Is an artificial pacemaker indicated?*

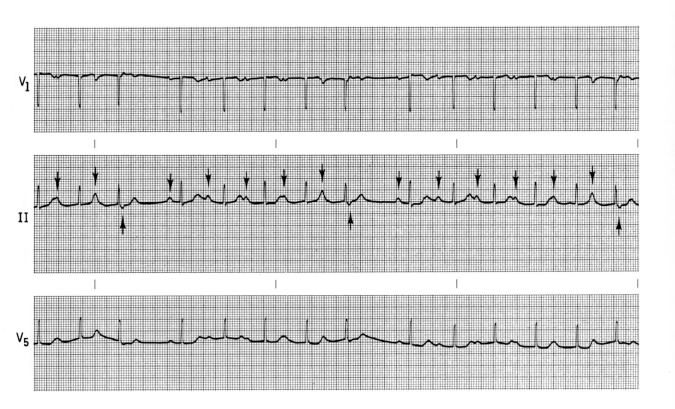

Case 96: Diagnosis

Downward arrows indicate sinus P waves. The underlying cardiac rhythm is sinus (atrial rate: 96 beats per minute, indicated by downward arrows) with Wenckebach A-V block. However, the characteristic features of the Wenckebach A-V block (see Case 37) are altered by the retrograde P wave (indicated by upward arrow) which occurs just before the occurrence of the expected blocked sinus P wave. This retrograde P wave (indicated by upward arrow) represents a reciprocal beat which is due to re-entry phenomenon in the A-V junction.

The reciprocal beat is commonly observed when there is a longitudinal dissociation in the A-V junction so that the degree of the prolonged refractoriness in the A-V junction differs considerably. Clinically, the reciprocal beats are not uncommon during Wenckebach A-V block. The reciprocal beat may appear as an isolated beat, such as seen in this case, but it may occur consecutively leading to reciprocating tachycardia (or re-entrant tachycardia).

In most cases, an artificial cardiac pacing is *not* indicated because the Wenckebach A-V block in recent diaphragmatic MI is a transient and self-limited electrophysiologic phenomenon (see Case 95).

Case 97

This ECG tracing was obtained from a 44-year-old man with a recent heart attack. He developed an irregular and slow heart rhythm soon after admission to the coronary care unit. He denied dizziness, near-syncope, or syncope, and his blood pressure was found to be stable (130/90 mm. Hg.).

1. *What is your cardiac rhythm diagnosis?*
2. *What is the underlying mechanism for altering the basic cardiac arrhythmia?*
3. *Is an artificial cardiac pacing indicated?*

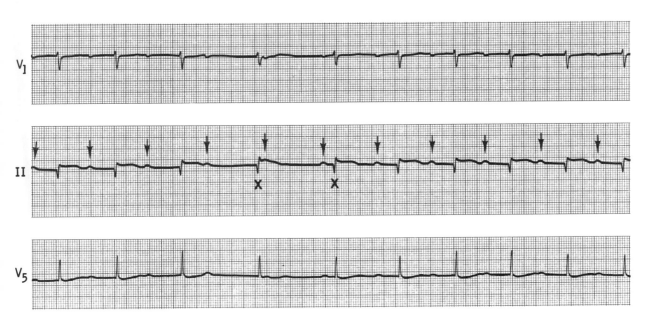

Case 97: Diagnosis

Arrows indicate sinus P waves. The underlying cardiac rhythm is sinus (atrial rate: 62 beats per minute) with slowly progressing Wenckebach A-V block associated with acute diaphragmatic MI. The characteristic features of Wenckebach A-V block (see Case 37) are altered in this tracing because of two consecutively occurring A-V junctional escape beats (marked X). Intermittent A-V junctional escape beats during Wenckebach A-V block is not uncommon.

An artificial cardiac pacing is *not* indicated under this circumstance as long as the patient is asymptomatic (e.g., no history of syncope or near-syncope) and there is no hemodynamic abnormality directly from the A-V block. Normal A-V conduction is usually restored spontaneously within hours or a few days in acute diaphragmatic MI in most cases.

Case 98

A 50-year-old man was admitted to the coronary care unit because of a sharp chest pain a few hours in duration. He was not taking any medication.

1. *What is your cardiac rhythm diagnosis?*
2. *What is the treatment of choice?*

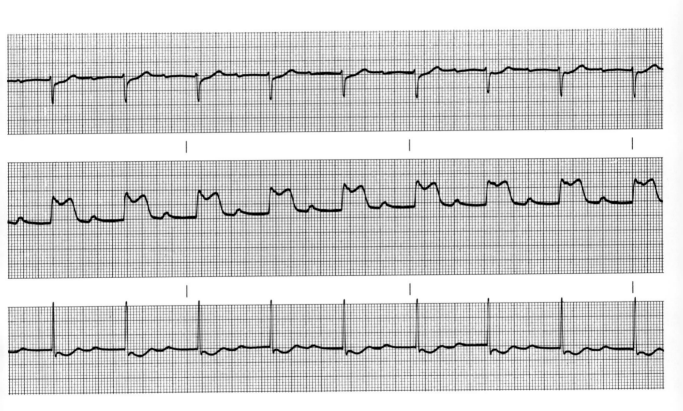

Case 98: Diagnosis

At a glance, the cardiac rhythm appears to be sinus rhythm with first degree A-V block. However, on a close observation, it becomes obvious that all other P waves are not conducted to the ventricles. Thus, the cardiac rhythm diagnosis is sinus tachycardia (atrial rate: 122 beats per minute) with 2:1 A-V block. Note that all other waves are superimposed on the last portion of the QRS complexes and an early portion of the S-T segment.

As described previously, 2:1 A-V block in recent diaphragmatic MI is usually a variant of Wenckebach A-V block (see Cases 94 and 95). Consequently, no treatment is indicated under this circumstance. Note marked S-T segment elevation in lead II, which indicates a very early sign of acute diaphragmatic MI.

Case 99

These rhythm strips were obtained in a coronary care unit from a patient with acute diaphragmatic MI. Leads II-a, b, and c are continuous.

1. *What is the ECG diagnosis?*
2. *What is the treatment of choice?*

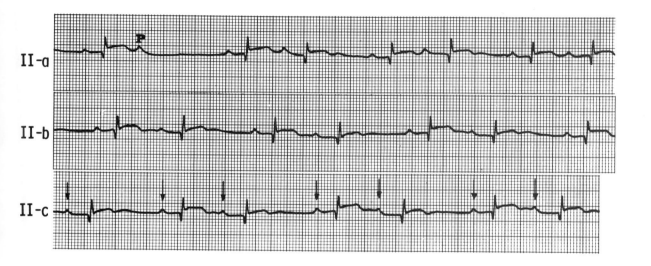

Case 99: Diagnosis

Arrows indicate sinus P waves. Long and short P-P cycles alternate throughout the tracing. The long P-P cycle is shorter than two P-P cycles. This regular irregularity of the P-P cycles represents 3:2 Wenckebach sino-atrial block. In addition, there is Wenckebach A-V conduction without actual blocked P waves throughout the tracing except for an early portion of lead II-a. A blocked P wave in Lead II-a is indicated by P. It is extremely interesting to observe that a characteristic feature of Wenckebach A-V block is altered by the 3:2 Wenckebach sino-atrial block (see Case 37).

An artificial pacemaker is indicated only when the patient is symptomatic (e.g., dizziness, near-syncope, or syncope) from the arrhythmia itself and/or when there is a significant hemodynamic abnormality (e.g., hypotension).

Case 100

A 72-year-old man was admitted to the coronary care unit because of a recent heart attack. On admission, he was found to have a very slow heart rate associated with unclear mental state and hypotension (85/60 mm. Hg.). He was not taking any medication.

1. *What is your cardiac rhythm diagnosis?*
2. *Is an artificial pacing indicated?*

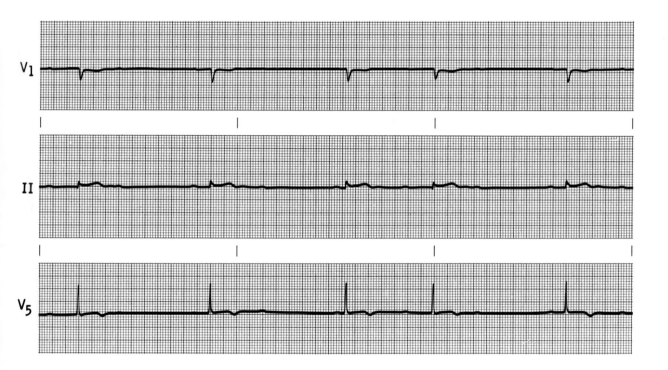

Case 100: Diagnosis

The underlying cardiac rhythm is sinus bradycardia (atrial rate: 54 beats per minute) with Wenckebach (Mobitz type I) A-V block and one A-V junctional escape beat (the 3rd QRS complex) producing a very slow ventricular rate (ventricular rate: 30–34 beats per minute). The characteristic features of Wenckebach A-V block (see Case 37) are slightly altered in this tracing because of occasional A-V junctional escape beats.

A temporary artificial packing is definitely indicated for this patient because of symptomatic A-V block associated with a hemodynamic abnormality due to a very slow ventricular rate. Wenckebach A-V block will disappear and normal A-V conduction will be restored within a few hours or days because the A-V block in acute diaphragmatic MI is usually transient in most cases.

As soon as the ventricular rate is increased to 72 beats per minute by an artificial pacing, his mental status improved and his blood pressure rose to a normal level (140/90 mm. Hg.).

Case 101

These ECG rhythm strips were obtained from a 59-year-old man with a recent heart attack.

1. *What is your ECG diagnosis?*
2. *What is the treatment of choice?*

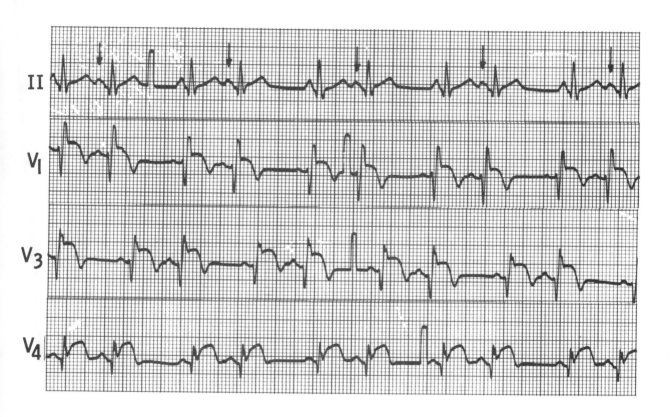

Case 101: Diagnosis

The underlying cardiac rhythm is sinus (rate: 86 beats per minute) but there are frequent atrial premature contractions (APCs, indicated by arrows) producing atrial bigeminy. The evidence of acute anterior MI and old diaphragmatic MI can be recognized without any difficulty. In addition, the diagnosis of incomplete right bundle branch block (RBBB) can be entertained.

By and large, no active treatment is indicated for APCs, but the patient should be observed closely for possible development of atrial tachyarrhythmias including atrial tachycardia, flutter, or fibrillation. In some cases, acute atrial tachyarrhythmias may signify atrial MI.

Case 102

These ECG rhythm strips were taken on a 48-year-old obese woman with a recent diaphragmatic MI. Leads II-a, b, and c are *not* continuous.

1. *What is your cardiac rhythm diagnosis?*
2. *What is the treatment of choice?*

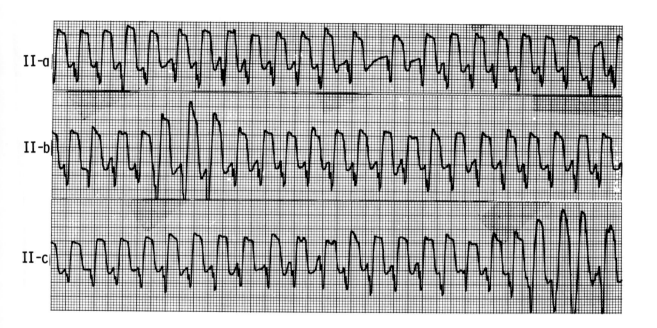

Case 102: Diagnosis

The cardiac rhythm is atrial fibrillation with very rapid ventricular response (ventricular rate: 160–180 beats per minute) and frequent aberrant ventricular conduction (the 5th, 6th, and 7th beats in lead II-b, and the last 4 beats in lead II-c). The S-T segment is markedly elevated throughout because of acute diaphragmatic MI.

The treatment of choice for atrial fibrillation with rapid ventricular response is rapid digitalization. When the clinical situation is extremely urgent, however, immediate application of direct current (DC) shock will be the treatment of choice.

Case 103

A 50-year-old man was admitted to the coronary care unit because of a recent heart attack. Upon admission, he was found to have a rapid heart rate.

1. *What is your ECG diagnosis?*
2. *What is the treatment of choice?*

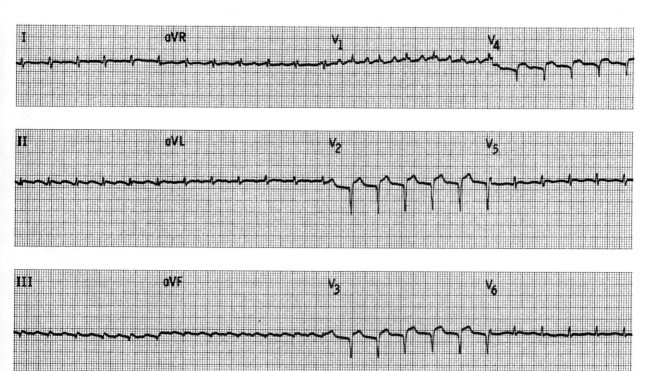

Case 103: Diagnosis

The cardiac rhythm is atrial flutter (atrial rate: 270 beats per minute) with 2:1 A-V response (ventricular rate: 135 beats per minute). The characteristic features of the atrial flutter waves (sawtooth appearance) are readily visible in many leads (e.g., leads II, III, and aVF).

The diagnosis of recent diaphragmatic as well as extensive anterior MI can be established on this ECG tracing without any difficulty. In addition, other ECG abnormalities include incomplete RBBB and low voltage of the QRS complexes.

As far as the therapeutic approach is concerned, the treatment of choice for atrial flutter with 2:1 A-V response is rapid digitalization. If the clinical situation is urgent, however, DC shock must be applied immediately. The effectiveness of DC shock for atrial flutter is nearly 100 percent.

Case 104

This ECG tracing was obtained from a 37-year-old man with a recent heart attack. His risk factors for coronary artery disease included mild diabetes mellitus, heavy cigarette smoking, and obesity. He was not taking any medication.

1. *What is your ECG diagnosis?*
2. *What is the treatment of choice?*

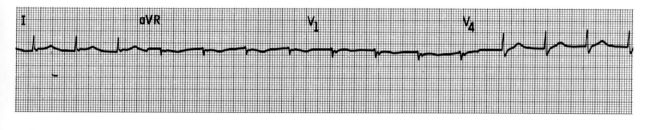

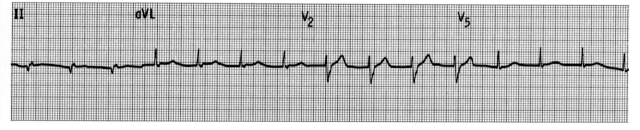

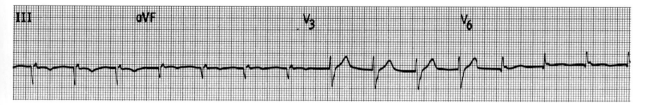

Case 104: Diagnosis

The cardiac rhythm is nonparoxysmal A-V junctional tachycardia with a rate of 84 beats per minute. Note that there is no discernible P wave and the ventricular cycle is precisely regular. Nonparoxysmal A-V junctional tachycardia is very common in recent diaphragmatic MI, and the arrhythmia is usually transient and self-limited. This patient suffered from recent diaphragmatic-lateral MI.

No treatment is indicated for nonparoxysmal A-V junctional tachycardia in recent diaphragmatic MI.

Case 105

A 48-year-old woman with coronary and hypertensive heart disease was complaining of palpitations. She was not taking any medication.

1. *What is your ECG diagnosis?*
2. *What is the treatment of choice?*

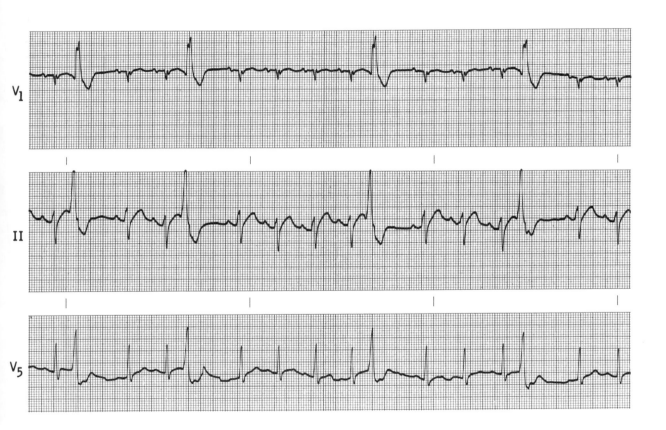

Case 105: Diagnosis

The underlying cardiac rhythm is sinus (rate: 98 beats per minute), but there are frequent ventricular premature contractures (VPCs) producing ventricular trigeminy and quadrigeminy. Note that the T waves of the preceding sinus beats are partially interrupted by the VPCs. This ECG finding is termed, the "R-on-T phenomenon" which often initiates ventricular fibrillation. The reason for this is that the threshold for the initiation of ventricular fibrillation is low during the vulnerable period of the ventricles corresponding approximately to the duration of the T waves. Therefore, aggressive treatment is indicated for VPCs with the R-on-T phenomenon. The VPCs in this ECG tracing are considered to be arising from the ventricular septum because the QRS complexes of the VPCs are predominantly positive (upright) in both the right and the left precordial leads (see Cases 77 and 79).

As far as the therapeutic approach is concerned, the drug of choice is intravenous injection of lidocaine (Xylocaine, 75–100 mg.) followed by intravenous infusion (1–5 mg. per minute). For long-term prophylactic purpose, one or more antiarrhythmic agents (e.g., quinidine, propranolol, procainamide) will be necessary for many cases under this circumstance.

Other ECG abnormalities include incomplete RBBB and left anterior hemiblock (the QRS axis is estimated to be −45 degrees).

Case 106

A 63-year-old man with a recent heart attack was admitted to the coronary care unit because of severe chest pain. Cardiac rhythm strips shown on this page (tracing A) were recorded soon after admission, whereas the rhythm strips shown on the next page (tracing B) were obtained immediately following the recording of the tracing A.

1. *What is the cardiac rhythm diagnosis of both tracings?*
2. *What is the best therapeutic approach?*

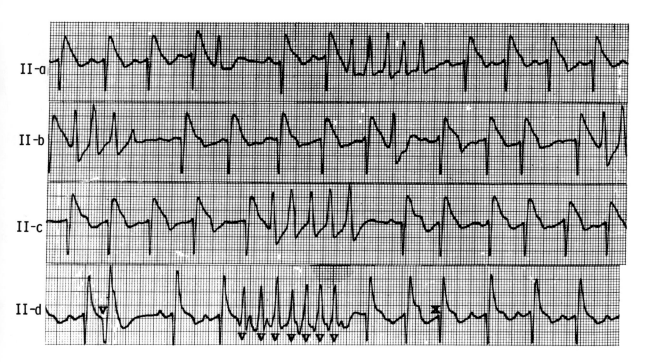

II-a

II-b

II-c

II-d

Case 106: Diagnosis

Tracing A: Leads II-a, b, c, and d are not continuous. The underlying cardiac rhythm is sinus (rate: 96 beats per minute) with first degree A-V block (P-R interval: 0.24 second). There are frequent multifocal VPCs with the R-on-T phenomenon, frequent ventricular group beats, and a short run of paroxysmal ventricular tachycardia (rate: 200–280 beats per minute, marked V). In addition, there are frequent APCs (marked X). The diagnosis of acute diaphragmatic MI is readily made. Almost immediately, the cardiac rhythm has transformed to ventricular fibrillation (tracing B).

Tracing B: Leads II-a, b, and c are continuous. The cardiac rhythm is ventricular fibrillation. As repeatedly stressed, ventricular fibrillation is easily provoked by VPCs when there is the R-on-T phenomenon because the threshold of ventricular fibrillation is markedly reduced during the T wave (the vulnerable period of the ventricles), especially in the presence of acute MI, as seen in this patient.

Management: Needless to say, the treatment of choice for ventricular fibrillation is immediate application of defibrillator (DC shock) with 200–400 wsec. If the first electric shock is ineffective, the shock treatment should be repeated with 400 wsec. without delay. In addition, all necessary cardiopulmonary resuscitative measures should be applied. It is uncommon to observe that the DC shock is effective to terminate ventricular fibrillation or tachycardia soon after intravenous injection of lidocaine (Xylocaine) in dosages of 50–100 mg. even if the first shock treatment (without lidocaine injection) may be ineffective.

When sinus rhythm is restored after termination of ventricular fibrillation, continuous intravenous infusion of lidocaine (1–5 mg. per minute) is definitely indicated at least for 24–48 hours (some patients require lidocaine for 1 week or more). In addition, one or more oral antiarrhythmic agents (e.g., quinidine, procainamide, Norpace, propranolol) may be required for months or even years if ventricular arrhythmias recur or persist. Frequent Holter monitor recordings are essential under these circumstances.

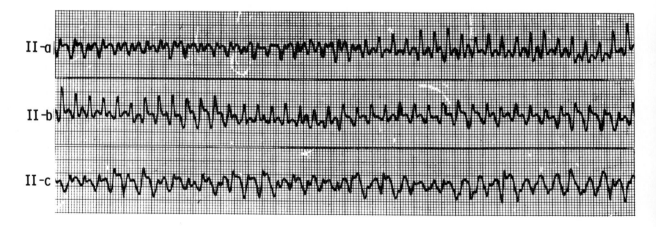

Case 107

This ECG tracing was taken on a 66-year-old man with acute diaphragmatic-lateral MI. Soon after admission to the coronary care unit, he developed bizarre QRS complexes without producing any symptom or hemodynamic abnormality. He was not taking any medication.

1. *What is your cardiac rhythm diagnosis?*
2. *What is the origin of the ectopic impulse formation for the production of this arrhythmia?*
3. *What is the treatment of choice?*

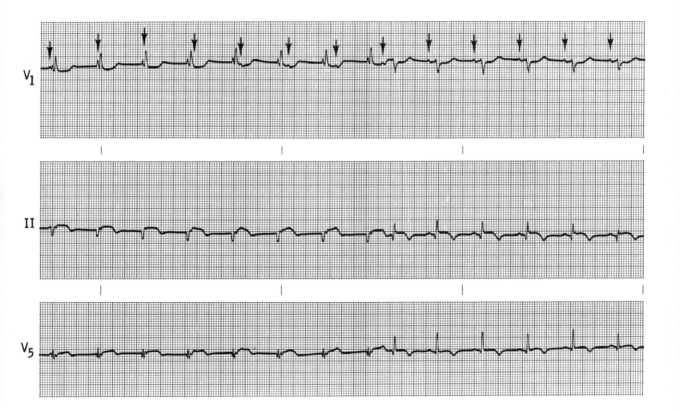

Case 107: Diagnosis

Arrows indicate sinus P waves. The underlying cardiac rhythm is sinus (rate: 80 beats per minute, indicated by arrows), but there are frequent bizarre QRS complexes causing incomplete A-V dissociation. The rate of the arrhythmia is very similar to that of sinus rhythm, and the QRS complexes exhibit incomplete RBBB pattern with marked left axis deviation. Thus, the arrhythmia is most likely arising from the posterior fascicle of the left bundle branch system—meaning fascicular tachycardia. The fascicular tachycardia is a form of nonparoxysmal ventricular tachycardia (accelerated ventricular rhythm or idioventricular tachycardia), which is not uncommon during an early phase (the first 24–72 hours) of acute MI (regardless of location of MI).

The fascicular tachycardia is usually transient in nature and self-limited. Accordingly, no treatment is indicated (see Case 86) for fascicular tachycardia.

Case 108

A 53-year-old man with a history of hypertension for many years was admitted to the coronary care unit because of severe chest pain of a few hours in duration. The only medication he was taking before admission was hydrochlorothiazide 50 mg. daily.

1. *What is your cardiac rhythm diagnosis?*
2. *What is the treatment of choice?*

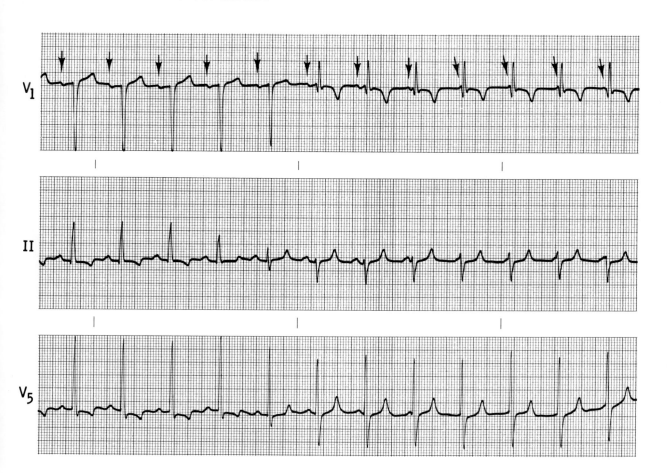

Case 108: Diagnosis

Arrows indicate P waves of sinus origin. The underlying cardiac rhythm is sinus (indicated by arrows; rate: 83 beats per minute) with first degree A-V block (P-R interval: 0.24 second). The diagnosis of the ectopic arrhythmia is a fascicular tachycardia (most likely originating from the left posterior fascicle; see Case 107), producing incomplete A-V dissociation.

As described previously (see Cases 86 and 107), no treatment is indicated for the fascicular tachycardia since the arrhythmia causes no symptom or any hemodynamic abnormality, and it is usually transient in nature.

Case 109

A 49-year-old man with Prinzmetal's angina was admitted to the coronary care unit because of increasing frequency and severity of chest pain. The cardiac rhythm strips shown in this page (tracing A) were obtained during chest pain, and the rhythm strips shown in the next page (tracing B) were recorded while the patient was treated with DC shock.

1. *What is the ECG diagnosis of the tracing A?*
2. *What is the cardiac rhythm diagnosis of the tracing B?*
3. *What is the best therapeutic approach?*

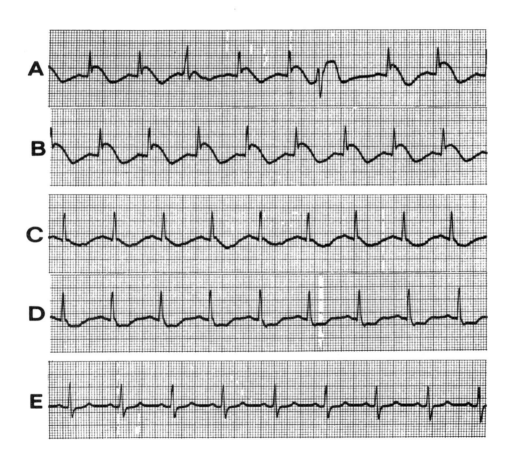

Case 109: Diagnosis

Tracing A: The rhythm strips A and B, and C and D are continuous in each given monitor lead. His cardiac events were recorded on 3 different occasions (A and B, C and D, and E) with a few minutes apart. The first 2 strips, A and B, reveal marked S-T segment elevation indicative of subepicardial injury (so-called "current injury"). The middle 2 ECG strips C and D disclose S-T segment depression, indicating subendocardial injury. The bottom strip E, which was recorded while the chest pain was almost subsided, shows near normal ECG.

His various S-T segment alterations during chest pain clearly indicate that coronary artery spasm may cause S-T segment elevation or depression, depending upon the involvement of a specific portion of the myocardium. Note a VPC in the rhythm strip A.

Tracing B: The cardiac monitor rhythm strips A, B, C, and D were recorded with a few seconds apart, whereas strips D and E are continuous. The initial cardiac arrhythmia is frequent VPCs leading to nonparoxysmal ventricular tachycardia (accelerated idioventricular rhythm; rate: 100 beats per minute—

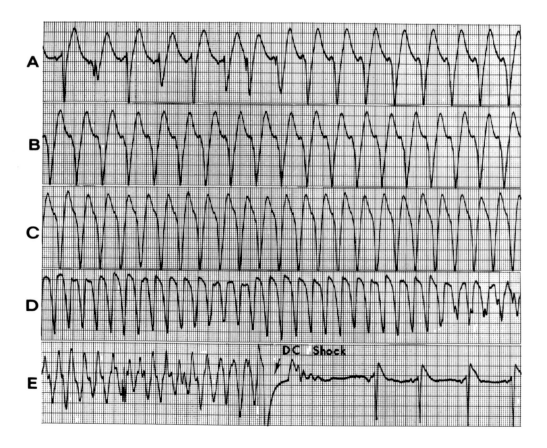

242

strip A). The rate of the tachycardia is progressively increased within a few seconds (strips B to D). As soon as the ventricular rate becomes faster than 220 beats per minute (strip D), he rapidly becomes unconscious, and finally ventricular fibrillation is produced (strip E). Fortunately, DC shock was effective in terminating ventricular fibrillation (indicated by arrow—strip E).

Management: In spite of continuous conventional therapy (e.g., nitroglycerin, propranolol, and all common antiarrhythmic agents), he developed many episodes of ventricular fibrillation with the same number as described as above. He consequently required DC shocks on many occasions.

It is rather unusual when nonparoxysmal ventricular tachycardia rapidly deteriorates to ventricular fibrillation because the former is nearly always self-limited and transient in nature. It can be said that this case report is an extremely rare clinical circumstance. In this patient, Nifedipine (a calcium-antagonist—still an investigative drug) was totally effective for his recurrent chest pain as well as the cardiac arrhythmia. The usual dosages of Nifedipine range from 40 to 160 mg. per day.

Coronary arteriography demonstrated 40% fixed stenosis of the circumflex artery, but 80% stenosis was produced by cold pressor test as a result of coronary artery spasm. It is not uncommon to observe coronary artery spasm in the presence of fixed coronary artery stenosis of varying degree.

Case 110

The electrocardiogram was obtained from a 56-year-old man with acute anterior MI. Leads II-a and b are not continuous.

What is your cardiac rhythm diagnosis?

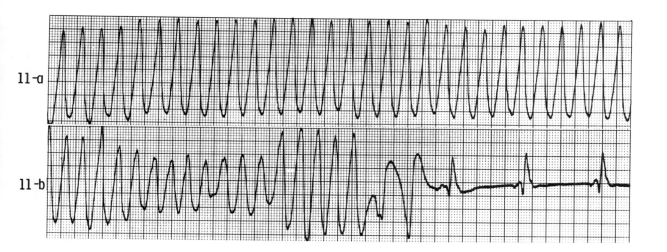

Case 110: Diagnosis

It is difficult to separate the S-T segment or T wave from the QRS complex in this ECG tracing. That is, the entire ECG complex appears to be a continuous loop. This kind of cardiac rhythm disorder is termed "ventricular flutter" (rate: 215 beats per minute), which has the same clinical significance as ventricular fibrillation (see Case 111). In other words, the cardiac output becomes negligible or even near zero during ventricular flutter or fibrillation. Therefore, ventricular flutter should be terminated immediately by DC shock. When the application of DC shock is delayed more than 4 minutes, irreversible brain damage is often unavoidable, even if the cardiac function is restored later. After the termination of ventricular flutter, continuous intravenous infusion (1–5 mg. per minute) of lidocaine (Xylocaine) is necessary for at least 24–72 hours in order to prevent the recurrence of ventricular tachyarrhythmias. Note that there are 3 near normal QRS complexes which may be the A-V junctional escape beats.

Case 111

These ECG rhythm strips were obtained from a 70-year-old woman with acute anterior MI. She developed cardiac arrest soon after arrival in the emergency room, and cardiopulmonary resuscitative measures were unsuccessful. Leads II-a, b, c, and d are not continuous.

What is your cardiac rhythm diagnosis?

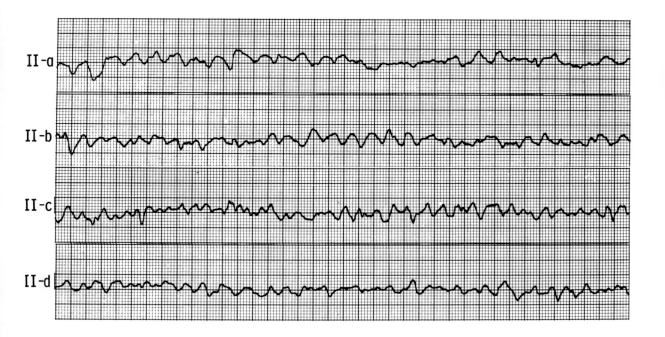

Case 111: Diagnosis

The cardiac rhythm is ventricular fibrillation, which is characterized by a chaotic ventricular cycle without discernible P waves, S-T segment, or T waves. Cardiac output during ventricular fibrillation is negligible or totally absent because the pumping action of the ventricles are ineffective. Immediate application of defibrillator with all available cardiopulmonary resuscitative measures will be, of course, the treatment of choice.

Case 112

A 63-year-old woman was admitted to the coronary care unit because of a recent heart attack. She developed bizarre and broad QRS complexes soon after admission.

1. *What is your ECG diagnosis?*
2. *Is a temporary cardiac pacemaker indicated?*
3. *Is a permanent pacemaker indicated?*

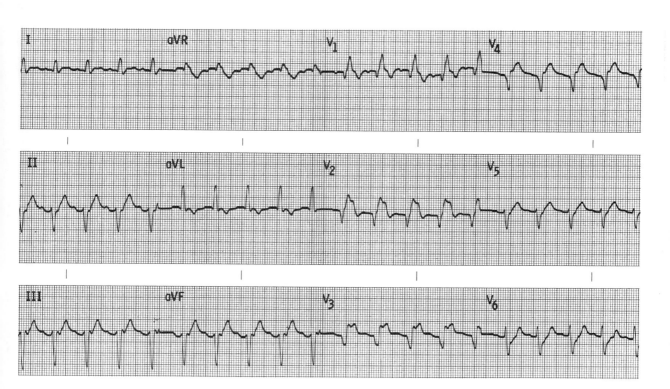

Case 112: Diagnosis

The cardiac rhythm is sinus tachycardia with a rate of 110 beats per minute. The diagnosis of acute bifascicular block (BFB) can be established because there is a combination of RBBB and left anterior hemiblock (LAHB) as a result of acute anteroseptal MI. The QRS axis is calculated to be −75 degrees. Of course, BFB is a form of incomplete bilateral bundle branch block (BBBB) (see Case 23).

The prophylactic artificial pacing is indicated for acute BFB as a result of a recent heart attack, usually involving the ventricular septum. A permanent artificial pacemaker is *not* indicated, however, under this circumstance as long as the patient does not develop a more advanced form of BBBB, particularly Mobitz type II A-V block (see Case 115) or complete A-V (infranodal) block, even transiently.

Case 113

A 67-year-old man with a history of hypertensive heart disease was admitted to the hospital because of severe chest pain associated with nausea, vomiting, and moderate dyspnea over the previous 2 hours.

What is the ECG diagnosis?

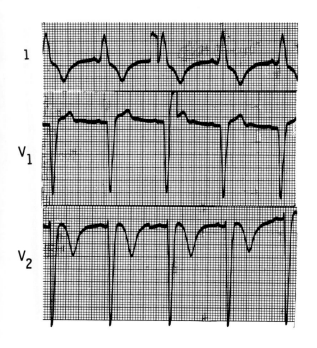

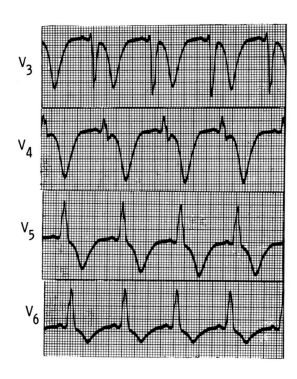

Case 113: Diagnosis

It is most difficult and at times impossible to diagnose MI in the presence of LBBB because the characteristic abnormal Q waves do not appear on the ECG. This is because the abnormal Q waves are concealed, since the alteration of the electrical forces during ventricular depolarization is predominantly influenced by the LBBB. Thus, the alterations of the S-T segment and T wave changes are most important for the diagnosis of MI in the presence of LBBB. The secondary S-T segment and T wave changes which always occur in uncomplicated LBBB will be altered by the primary T wave change. Note deeply and symmetrically inverted T waves involving many leads. Remember that a pure LBBB characteristically discloses biphasic to slightly inverted (*not* symmetrically) T waves in the left precordial leads (leads I, aVL, and V_{4-6}) as the secondary T wave change (see Case 21).

A value of the prophylactic artificial pacing for LBBB (either pre-existing or new onset) associated with acute MI is not fully established.

Case 114

A 61-year-old man was admitted to the hospital because of severe chest pain over the previous 2 hours and expired the following day.

What is the ECG diagnosis?

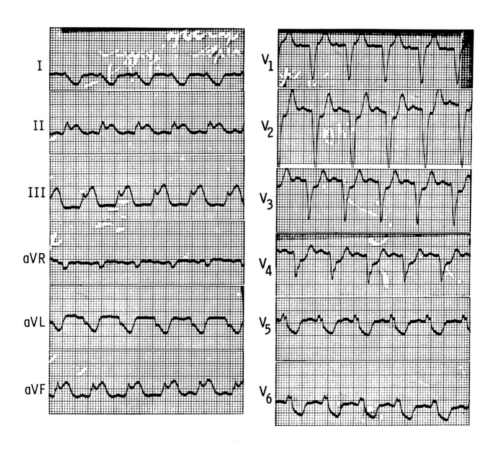

Case 114: Diagnosis

The basic rhythm is sinus with a rate of 100 beats per minute. The QRS complexes are wide due to LBBB. In addition, the S-T segment is markedly elevated in leads II, III, and aVF, indicating acute diaphragmatic subepicardial injury, which is most likely an early change of acute diaphragmatic MI. Typical secondary S-T segment and T wave changes which are always present in uncomplicated LBBB are absent here because of coexisting acute MI. The diagnosis of MI in the presence of LBBB is often difficult, and at times impossible. Under these circumstances, an alteration of the S-T segment and/or T wave changes may be the only evidence of MI.

In addition, the S-T segment is markedly and horizontally depressed in V_{2-4}, and this ECG finding most likely represents posterior subepicardial injury—an early sign of acute posterior MI. Remember that the S-T segment in these anterior precordial leads (V_{1-4}) in a pure LBBB is usually elevated rather than depressed.

Case 115

This electrocardiogram was obtained from a 72-year-old woman who has been suffering from lightheadedness. MI occurred 6 months ago in this patient, but her recovery was uneventful. She was not taking any drug.

1. *What is your cardiac rhythm diagnosis?*
2. *Is artificial pacing indicated?*

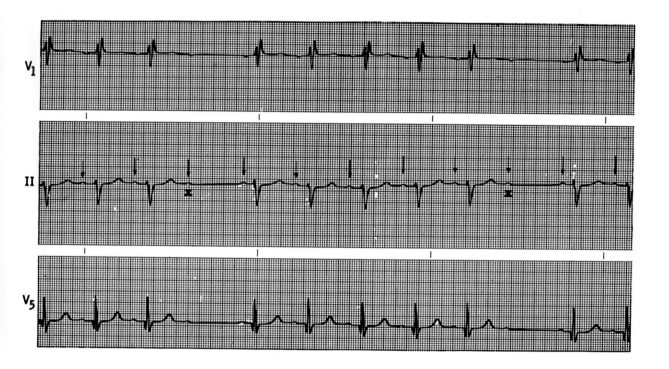

Case 115: Diagnosis

Arrows indicate sinus P waves. The cardiac rhythm reveals sinus rhythm (indicated by arrows; atrial rate: 64 beats per minute) with first degree A-V block (P-R interval 0.24 second) and intermittent Mobitz type-II A-V block. Note that the P-R intervals remain constant in all conducted beats until a blocked P wave (marked X) occurs. Thus, the long R-R interval (ventricular pause) which contains a blocked P wave (marked X) is exactly 2 times the basic P-P cycles. These ECG findings are characteristic features of Mobitz type-II A-V block which represents infranodal block. It is well documented that Mobitz type-II A-V block is a precursor of complete A-V block due to complete trifascicular block.

In Mobitz type-II A-V block, the QRS complexes almost always demonstrate LBBB or RBBB or a BFB (see Chapter 2). In this case, a combination of first degree A-V block with intermittent Mobitz type-II A-V block and a BFB [RBBB plus left anterior hemiblock (LAHB)] represents incomplete trifascicular block (TFB) (incomplete BBBB; see Chapter 2 and Case 23).

This patient had suffered from extensive anterior MI (except septum) 6 months ago, and abnormal Q waves are present in leads V_2 through V_6—only 3 leads are shown here.

She underwent permanent artificial pacemaker (demand unit) implantation. No further episode of lightheadedness was observed thereafter.

It should be remembered that Mobitz type-II A-V block is a form of incomplete TFB and the block is irreversible—infranodal block.

Case 116

This ECG tracing was obtained from a 62-year-old man with a recent heart attack. The prophylactic artificial pacemaker was inserted because he developed a very slow heart rhythm soon after admission.

1. *What is your ECG diagnosis?*
2. *What is the underlying cardiac arrhythmia which required the prophylactic pacing?*

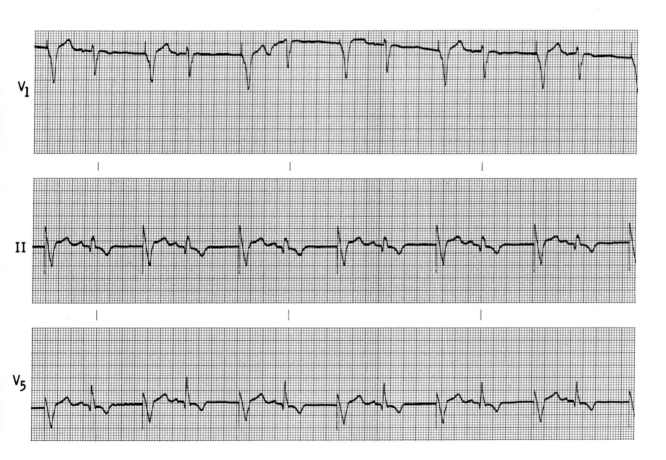

Case 116: Diagnosis

The underlying cardiac rhythm is markedly slow sinus bradycardia with a rate of 38 beats per minute. In addition, there are demand pacemaker-induced QRS complexes which occur on every other beat. This type of bigeminal rhythm is termed "escape-bigeminy," and specifically, the arrhythmia shown in this tracing is termed "pacemaker-escape-bigeminy."

It is a well known fact that marked sinus bradycardia is not uncommon in recent diaphragmatic MI. In this ECG tracing, the diagnosis of recent diaphragmatic-lateral MI can be made without any difficulty.

When markedly slow sinus bradycardia persists and is drug-resistant, SSS should be suspected. When the diagnosis of SSS is established, permanent artificial pacing should be considered (see Chapter 1).

Case 117

The prophylactic artificial pacing was inserted because a 48-year-old man developed acute BFB as a result of acute extensive anterior MI.

1. *What is your ECG diagnosis?*
2. *What is the reason the demand ventricular pacemaker takes over the ventricular activity from time to time?*

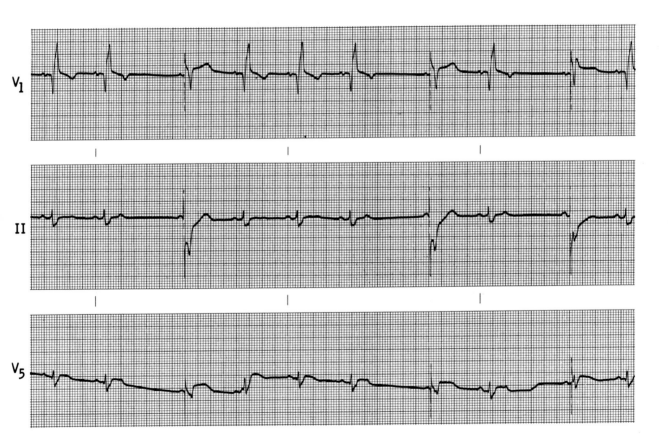

Case 117: Diagnosis

The underlying cardiac rhythm is sinus with a rate of 72 beats per minute. The demand ventricular pacemaker takes over the ventricular activity whenever a ventricular pause is longer than the preset pacemaker escape interval. Upon close observation, frequent nonconducted (blocked) APCs can be recognized, and the blocked APCs are responsible for the production of the ventricular pauses. The blocked APCs are superimposed to the T waves of the preceding beats.

The BFB in this ECG tracing consists of RBBB and LAHB (see Case 23), and the finding is, of course, a form of partial BBBB (see Case 23). Prophylactic artificial pacing is indicated for acute BFB due to anterior MI.

It can be said that a blocked APC is the most common cause of a ventricular pause.

chapter 6

Cardiac Arrhythmias Related to Wolff-Parkinson-White Syndrome

Case 118

This ECG tracing was obtained from a 56-year-old woman as a part of an annual medical check-up. She had experienced chest tightness on several occasions and frequent rapid heart actions. She was not taking any medication, however.

1. *What is your ECG diagnosis?*
2. *What is the fundamental mechanism for producing this ECG finding?*

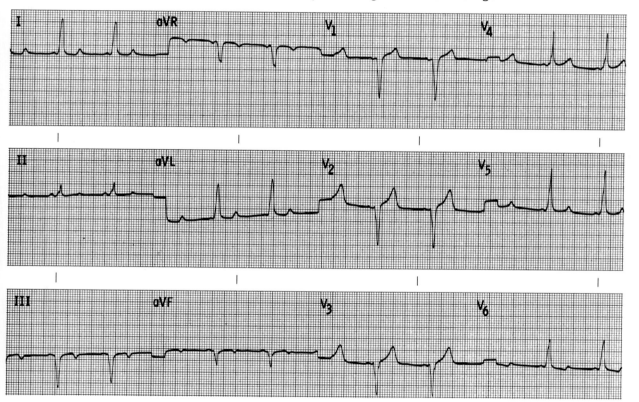

Case 118: Diagnosis

The cardiac rhythm is sinus with a rate of 64 beats per minute. The diagnosis of Wolff-Parkinson-White (WPW) syndrome is established on the basis of a short P-R interval with a broad QRS complex due to a delta wave (the initial slurring of the QRS complex) associated with secondary T wave change in the left precordial leads.

The initial slurring of the QRS complex is often called a "delta wave" and is considered to be the result of a premature activation of a portion of the ventricles as a result of an anomalous A-V conduction via an accessory pathway.

WPW syndrome is customarily classified into 2 types—type A and type B. WPW syndrome shown in this ECG tracing is type B because the QRS complex is primarily negative (downward) in leads V_{1-3} and upright (positive) in leads V_{4-6}. In type B WPW syndrome, the premature activation takes place in a

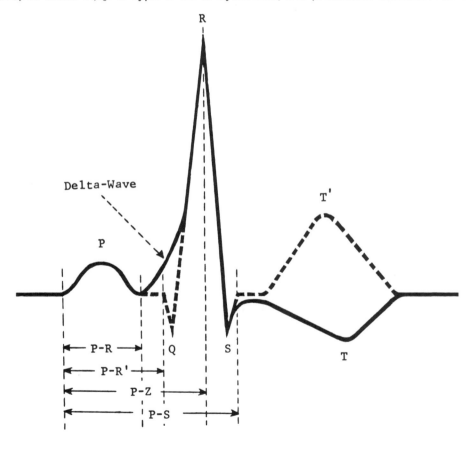

DIAGRAM : WOLFF-PARKINSON-WHITE SYNDROME

portion of the right ventricle via an anomalous pathway which is located in the right ventricle. Conversely, in type A WPW syndrome, the premature activation occurs in a portion of the left ventricle so that the QRS complexes are primarily upright (positive) in the right precordium and downward (negative) in the left precordium. When the accessory pathway is situated in a posterior portion of the left ventricle, the QRS complexes will be upright in all precordial leads—a variant of type A WPW syndrome.

In general, on a superficial examination, type A WPW syndrome resembles right bundle branch block (RBBB) (see Cases 119, 124, and 126) whereas type B WPW syndrome (as shown in this tracing) simulates left bundle branch block (LBBB).

The fundamental mechanism underlying this unique ECG finding in the WPW syndrome is diagrammatically illustrated. The uninterrupted line indicates the anomalous conduction in the WPW syndrome; the dotted line, normal condition. The P-R and P-R' intervals are A-V conduction time in the WPW syndrome and normal conduction, respectively. The P-R interval is shorter than the P-R' interval as a result of a delta wave. Note that the P-Z and P-S intervals are constant during anomalous and normal conduction. The T wave in the WPW syndrome is inverted because of a secondary T wave change.

The most important clinical significance of the WPW syndrome is the extremely high incidence (50–75%) of various supraventricular tachyarrhythmias. This patient was found to have frequent episodes of reciprocating tachycardia that required propranolol (Inderal) therapy.

Another ECG abnormality in this ECG tracing is inverted T waves in leads III and aVF indicative of diaphragmatic myocardial ischemia. Remember that the secondary T wave change usually shows that the direction of the T wave is opposite to that of the QRS complex.

Case 119

This ECG tracing was taken on a 43-year-old woman with many episodes of palpitations. She was not taking any medication regularly.

1. *What is your ECG diagnosis?*
2. *What is the best approach to document her rapid heart action?*

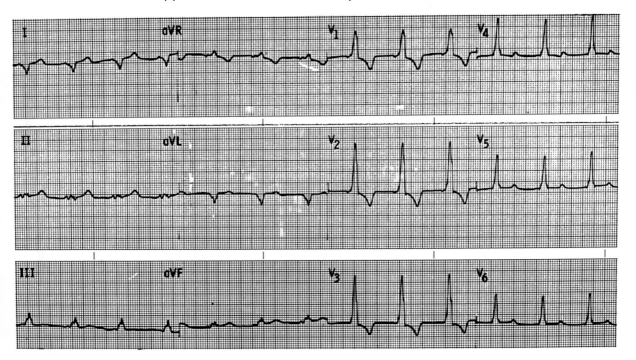

Case 119: Diagnosis

The cardiac rhythm is sinus with a rate of 73 beats per minute. The P waves are not clearly visible in most areas because the P-R interval is very short due to a broad delta wave. Thus, the diagnosis of WPW syndrome, type A can be readily made.

The ECG finding closely simulates RBBB, LBBB or even bilateral bundle branch block (BBBB) (see Chapter 2). In addition, high lateral myocardial infarction is simulated in view of Q-S waves in leads I and aVL by virtue of negative (downward) delta wave in these leads.

The best diagnostic approach to document her arrhythmia is, of course, frequent Holter monitor recordings.

Case 120

These Holter monitor ECG rhythm strips were obtained from a 32-year-old man with palpitations. On physical examination, he was found to be healthy and his 12-lead ECG was entirely within normal limits. The strips A, B, and C are not continuous.

What is your ECG diagnosis?

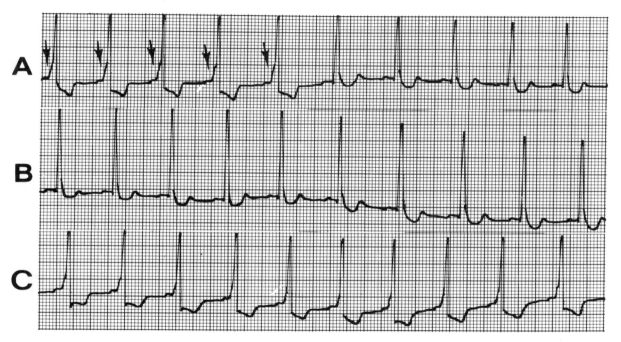

Case 120: Diagnosis

The cardiac rhythm is sinus with a rate of 82 beats per minute. It is obvious that there are 2 kinds of QRS complexes. This ECG finding represents intermittent WPW syndrome (indicated by arrows). Although the episode of specific tachyarrhythmias is *not* recorded on the Holter monitor ECG, the underlying WPW syndrome which frequently causes various rapid heart actions is documented. The Holter monitor recording is ordered again in this patient in order to document the tachyarrhythmia.

Case 121

These ECG rhythm strips were recorded on a 7-week-old infant. Cardiac consultation was requested because of the electrocardiographic abnormality. The baby was free of any symptom from cardiac viewpoint. Leads I-a and b and lead V_1-a and b are continuous in each given lead.

1. *What is your ECG diagnosis?*
2. *What is the best therapeutic approach?*

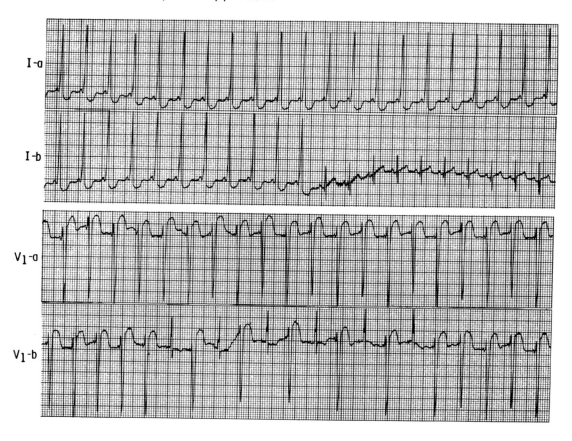

Case 121: Diagnosis

The cardiac rhythm is sinus tachycardia with a rate of 150 beats per minute. It is obvious that there are 2 kinds of the QRS complexes. This ECG finding is due to intermittent Wolff-Parkinson-White syndrome.

Intermittent WPW syndrome superficially resembles frequent ventricular premature contractures (VPCs) and paroxysmal ventricular tachycardia. In addition, intermittent LBBB is closely simulated.

No treatment is indicated for this infant as long as there is no history of documented ectopic tachyarrhythmias. As stressed repeatedly, paroxysmal supraventricular tachyarrhythmias are very common in all individuals with WPW syndrome (see Cases 123, 124, 125, and 126). Therefore, periodic medical check-ups are highly recommended.

Case 122

A 24-year-old, apparently healthy man was referred to a cardiologist for the evaluation of frequent rapid heart actions. The Holter monitor ECG was obtained in order to determine the nature of the paroxysmal rapid heart actions. His 12-lead ECG was entirely within normal limits (not shown here).

1. *What is the ECG diagnosis?*
2. *How would you treat this patient?*

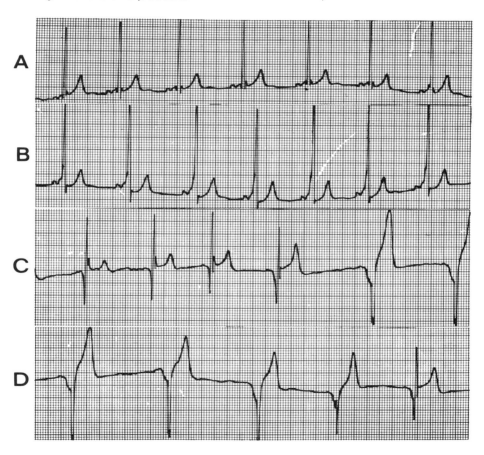

Case 122: Diagnosis

The rhythm strips A through D are not continuous. The Holter monitor ECG reveals sinus arrhythmia with periods of marked sinus bradycardia (rate: 42–57 beats per minute). Unfortunately, no episode of the paroxysmal rapid heart action was recorded on the Holter monitor ECG. The most interesting finding, however, was the WPW syndrome, with multiple anomalous A-V conductions causing various QRS complex configurations.

Later, a paroxysmal supraventricular (reciprocating) tachycardia was documented by repeating the Holter monitor ECG (not shown here) on this patient.

When documentation of the nature of the paroxysmal tachyarrhythmia is not possible on repeated Holter monitor recordings, small amounts of oral propranolol (Inderal) (10–30 mg., 3–4 times daily) should be tried, since in reciprocating tachycardia with a normal QRS complex, the most common tachycardia in the WPW syndrome, this agent is the drug of choice.

The fundamental mechanism responsible for the ECG abnormality in the WPW syndrome has been described (Case 118). The diagrams explaining the mechanisms responsible for the tachyarrhythmias in the WPW syndrome are found elsewhere (see Case 123).

A 47-year-old woman was referred to the cardiac clinic for evaluation of her frequent palpitations. Although her 12-lead ECG demonstrated a type A WPW syndrome on several occasions (not shown here), her tachyarrhythmias had never been documented. Thus, a Holter monitor ECG was ordered.

1. *What is the cardiac rhythm diagnosis?*
2. *What is the fundamental mechanism underlying the various tachyarrhythmias in the WPW syndrome?*
3. *What is the drug of choice?*

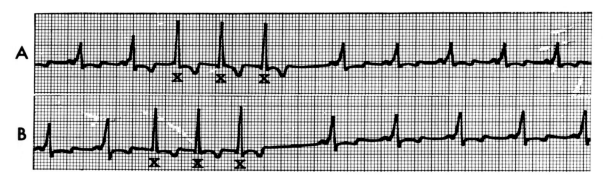

Case 123: Diagnosis

Strips A and B are not continuous. The Holter monitor recording demonstrates three group beats with "normal" QRS morphology (X) during sinus rhythm with anomalous (WPW syndrome) A-V conduction. The implication was that group beats with a normal QRS morphology represent re-entry beats that conduct, in retrograde fashion, through the bypass tract, and in antegrade fashion, through the A-V junction. The P waves, however, are not clearly seen in group beats. In this patient, recurrent reciprocating tachycardias were treated with propranolol (Inderal). It has been shown that propranolol is the drug of choice in the treatment as well as the prevention of reciprocating tachycardia with normal QRS complexes in the WPW syndrome.

The fundamental mechanism underlying reciprocating tachycardia in the WPW syndrome is described as follows:

Diagram (Part I) illustrating the mechanism of a reciprocating tachycardia with a normal QRS complex in the WPW syndrome. In A, the atrial premature impulse (A) is conducted to the A-V node (N), but the atrial premature impulse is blocked in the anomalous pathway. The atrial premature impulse is then conducted to both ventricles via the bundle branch system (A). In B, the atrial impulse is conducted to the atria, in retrograde fashion, to produce an inverted P wave. In C, the impulse is conducted clockwise to produce a reciprocating (re-entry) cycle; the same cycle may repeat indefinitely. Note that the QRS complex during tachycardia is normal. Key: S, sinus node; d, delta wave; P, inverted P wave.

Diagram (Part II) illustrating a reciprocating tachycardia with anomalous conduction in the WPW syndrome. The re-entry cycle is counterclockwise, which is exactly the reverse of that shown in the Part I diagram.

It has been shown that a reciprocating tachycardia is the most common tachyarrhythmia associated with the WPW syndrome, and the majority of cases show normal QRS complexes. Less commonly, atrial fibrillation (AF) may be observed; atrial flutter is extremely rare in the WPW syndrome. In both AF and atrial flutter, the QRS complexes are almost always bizarre because anomalous A-V conduction and/or aberrant ventricular conduction occur as the result of the extremely rapid ventricular rate (see cases 124–126).

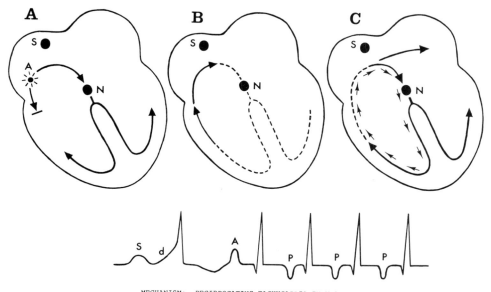

MECHANISM: RECIPROCATING TACHYCARDIA IN W P W SYNDROME

PART I: NORMAL QRS COMPLEX

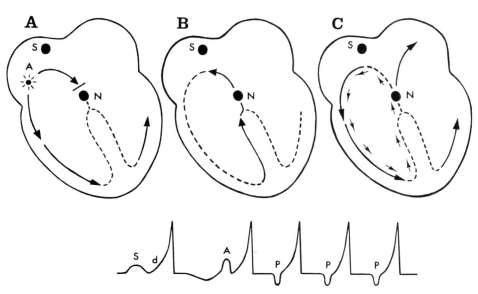

MECHANISM: RECIPROCATING TACHYCARDIA IN W P W SYNDROME

PART II: ABNORMAL QRS COMPLEX (ANOMALOUS A-V CONDUCTION)

A 40-year-old woman was seen in the emergency room because of extremely rapid heart rate. She complained of palpitations associated with weakness. She told an emergency room physician that she had experienced frequent palpitations since childhood. She was not taking any drugs.

1. *What is the cardiac rhythm diagnosis during rapid heart action?*
2. *What is the treatment of choice?*
3. *What is the 12-lead ECG diagnosis after termination of the rapid heart action?*

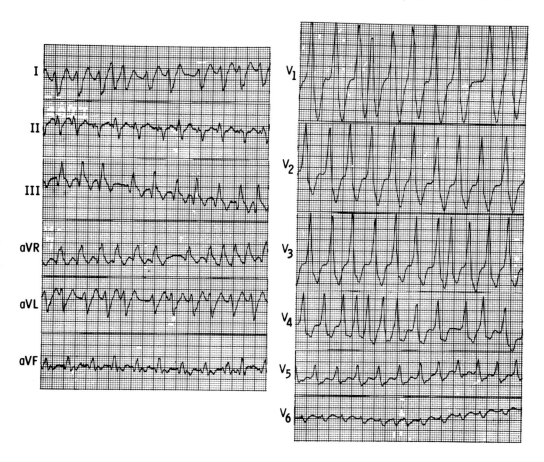

Case 124: Diagnosis

Tracing A—12-lead ECG (during paroxysm): The cardiac rhythm is AF with anomalous A-V conduction, because of the WPW syndrome and an extremely rapid ventricular rate (rate: 160–250 beats per minute). The ECG finding closely mimics ventricular tachycardia.

When the clinical situation is extremely urgent, direct current shock should be applied immediately. Otherwise, the treatment of choice is an intravenous injection of lidocaine (Xylocaine), which can block conduction through the accessory pathway in the WPW syndrome. Quinidine or procainamide are equally effective for prophylaxis. The mechanism that produces tachyarrhythmias in the WPW syndrome has been described in detail elsewhere (see Case 123).

Tracing B—12-lead ECG (after paroxysm): The cardiac rhythm is sinus with a rate of 100 beats per minute. The diagnosis of the WPW syndrome, type A, is readily made on the basis of short P-R intervals with broad upright QRS complexes in all precordial leads, as a result of delta waves (see Case 118).

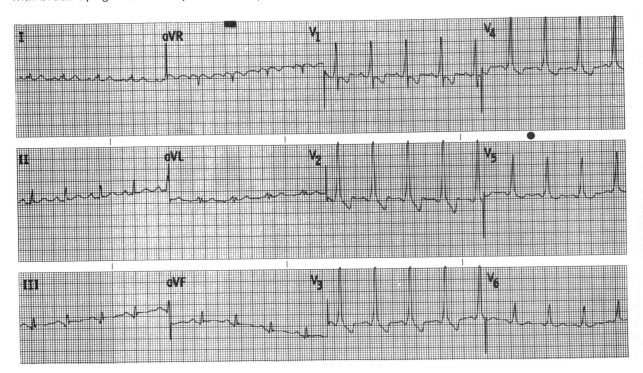

Case 125

A 44-year-old apparently healthy woman was brought to the emergency room because of a very rapid heart action. She gave a history of similar episodes in the past, but she was not taking any medication regularly.

1. *What is your ECG diagnosis?*
2. *What is the best therapeutic approach?*

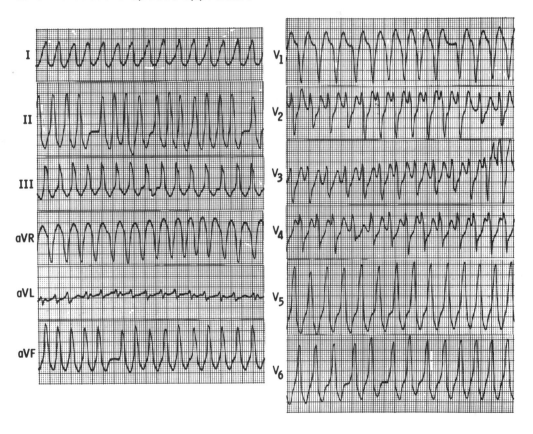

Case 125: Diagnosis

The cardiac rhythm is AF with broad QRS complexes due to anomalous A-V conduction in WPW syndrome, type B. Ventricular tachycardia is closely simulated.

The best therapeutic approach under this clinical circumstance has been described previously (see Case 124).

By and large, AF or atrial flutter associated with WPW syndrome is much more difficult to treat compared with reciprocating tachycardia (see Case 123), although the latter is much more common. If AF or atrial flutter associated with WPW syndrome becomes refractory to the conventional drug therapy, various investigative drugs (e.g., amiodarone) should be tried. When the tachyarrhythmia persists in spite of all available drugs, the surgical approach (e.g., ligation of the accessory pathway) has to be considered in selected cases.

Case 126

A 24-year-old healthy man developed rapid heart action; he had suffered from similar episodes previously. He was not taking any drugs.

1. *What is the cardiac rhythm diagnosis during rapid heart action?*
2. *What is the disorder underlying the rapid heart action?*
3. *What is the treatment of choice?*

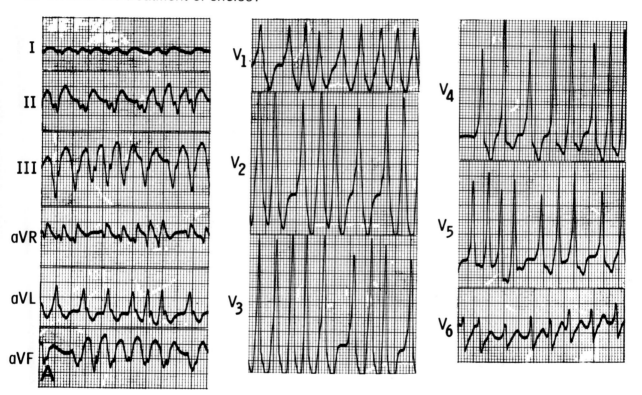

Case 126: Diagnosis

Tracing A—12-lead ECG (during paroxysm): The cardiac rhythm appears to be ventricular tachycardia or even ventricular fibrillation (VF). However, the correct diagnosis is AF with anomalous A-V conduction due to WPW syndrome, type A. The ventricular rate is extremely rapid (180–300 beats per minute), and the QRS configuration is broad and bizarre. The diagnosis of WPW syndrome, type A, is obvious during sinus rhythm.

The treatment of choice is the immediate application of direct current shock (100–200 W-sec.). When the clinical situation is not urgent, intravenous injection of lidocaine (Xylocaine) (50–100 mg.) is the treatment of choice. For prophylaxis, oral quinidine or procainamide (Pronestyl) are the drugs of choice.

Propranolol (Inderal) is totally ineffective in such cases. Digitalis is not only ineffective, but it also can enhance the anomalous A-V conduction, leading to deterioration of the patient. In fact, this patient

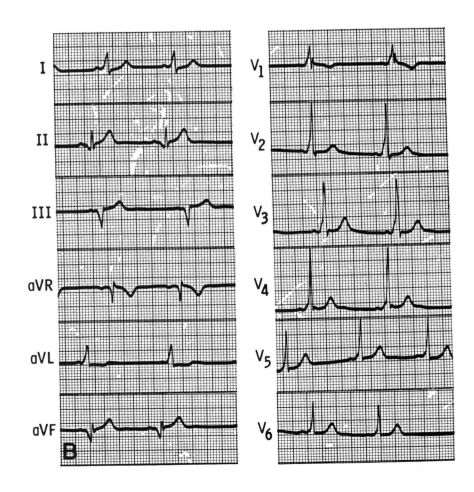

developed a true VF soon after the administration of digitalis, but fortunately a defibrillator was used immediately and sinus rhythm was restored.

Tracing B—12-lead ECG (after paroxysm): The cardiac rhythm is sinus arrhythmia with a rate of 55–70 beats per minute. The diagnosis of the WPW syndrome, type A, is obvious (see Case 118). Note a pseudodiaphragmatic and posterior myocardial infarction pattern during sinus rhythm because of the type A WPW syndrome.

Chapter 7

Digitalis-Induced Arrhythmias

Case 127

This ECG tracing was obtained from a 64-year-old man with chronic congestive heart failure due to hypertensive heart disease. Digitalis toxicity was suspected.

1. *What is your cardiac rhythm diagnosis?*
2. *What is the treatment of choice?*

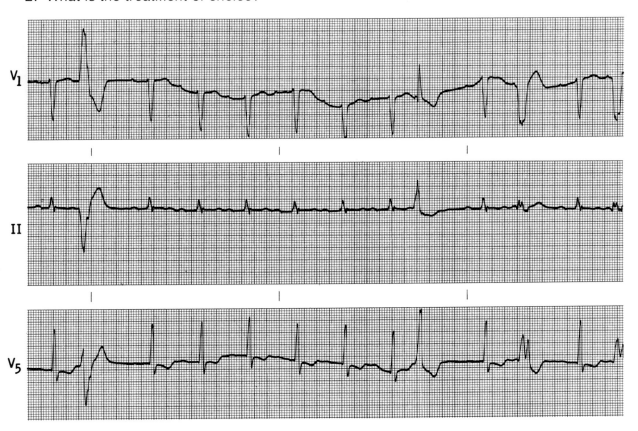

Case 127: Diagnosis

The underlying cardiac rhythm is sinus (rate: 78 beats per minute) with first degree A-V block (P-R interval: 0.28 second). It should be noted that there are 3 kinds of bizarre and broad QRS complexes—multifocal ventricular premature contractions (VPCs) showing areas of ventricular bigeminy.

Multifocal VPCs and ventricular bigeminy have been considered a hallmark of digitalis intoxication (toxicity) for many decades. A-V block of various degrees is also common in digitalis toxicity because the drug has a depressive action in the A-V junction leading to prolongation of the refractory period in the A-V node. Wenckebach A-V block is probably the most common A-V conduction disturbance in digitalis toxicity (see Cases 61, 128, 131, and 142).

Needless to say, the treatment of choice for digitalis-induced arrhythmias is immediate discontinuation of digitalis. When the serum potassium is found to be low, supplementary potassium administration is beneficial. In addition, diphenylhydantoin (Dilantin) is very effective for various digitalis-induced tachyarrhythmias, particularly those ventricular in origin.

Case 128

A 51-year-old hypertensive woman was admitted to the intermediate cardiac care unit because she developed a rapid heart action during a maintenance oral (0.25 mg. daily) digoxin therapy for chronic congestive heart failure.

What is your cardiac rhythm diagnosis?

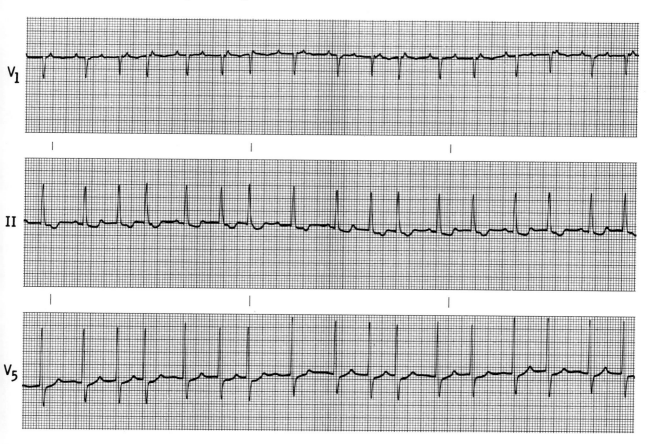

Case 128: Diagnosis

The ventricular cycle reveals a rather irregularity—meaning *not* grossly irregular—but the atrial cycle is regular. Thus, the cardiac rhythm diagnosis is atrial tachycardia (atrial rate: 160 beats per minute) with Wencekebach (Mobitz type I) A-V block of 4:3 and 3:2 A-V conduction ratios. Note that the P-R intervals progressively lengthen until a blocked P wave occurs. At the same time, the R-R intervals (the ventricular cycles) progressively shorten until a blocked P wave occurs. The mechanism of Wenckebach A-V block has been fully described previously (see Case 37). Paroxysmal atrial tachycardia (PAT) with Wenckebach A-V block may be misdiagnosed as atrial fibrillation on the basis of the irregular ventricular cycle if the reader fails to recognize the ectopic P waves.

Atrial tachycardia with Wenckebach A-V block has been termed "PAT with block" by some investigators. This arrhythmia is not as common in digitalis toxicity as previously thought. If PAT with block is found in any individual, however, the diagnosis of digitalis toxicity is almost certain—meaning almost pathognomonic feature of digitalis toxicity. At times, atrial tachycardia with Wenckebach A-V block may transform to atrial tachycardia with 2:1 A-V block from time to time in the same patient with digitalis intoxication (see Case 129).

Her serum digoxin level was reported to be significantly elevated (3.2 ng./ml.). The therapeutic serum digoxin level ranged from 1.0 to 2.5 ng./ml.

Digitalis toxicity was suspected on a 39-year-old man with idiopathic cardiomyopathy.

What is your cardiac rhythm diagnosis?

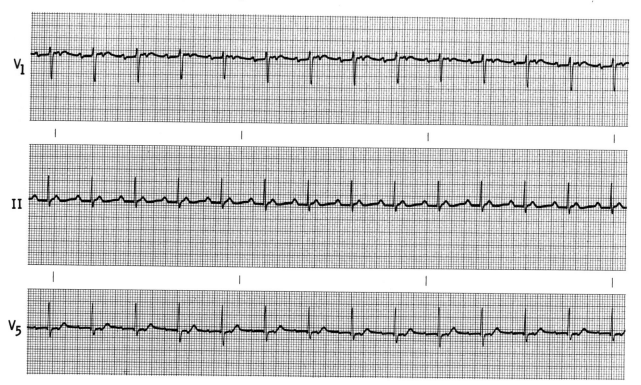

Case 129: Diagnosis

The cardiac rhythm is atrial tachycardia (atrial rate: 176 beats per minute) with 2:1 A-V block (ventricular rate: 88 beats per minute). Note that every other P wave is conducted to the ventricles and the cardiac cycle is precisely regular. If every other P wave is not recognized—common practice—the cardiac rhythm may be easily misdiagnosed as normal sinus rhythm.

As discussed previously, atrial tachycardia with 2:1 A-V block is usually a variant of atrial tachycardia with Wenckebach A-V block in digitalis intoxication (see Case 128). Digitalis toxicity is relatively common in patients with cardiomyopathy.

Case 130

A 56-year-old man with cardiomyopathy was examined in the cardiac clinic because he developed a cardiac arrhythmia during chronic digitalization.

1. *What is your cardiac rhythm diagnosis?*
2. *Which cardiac chamber enlargement is diagnosed?*

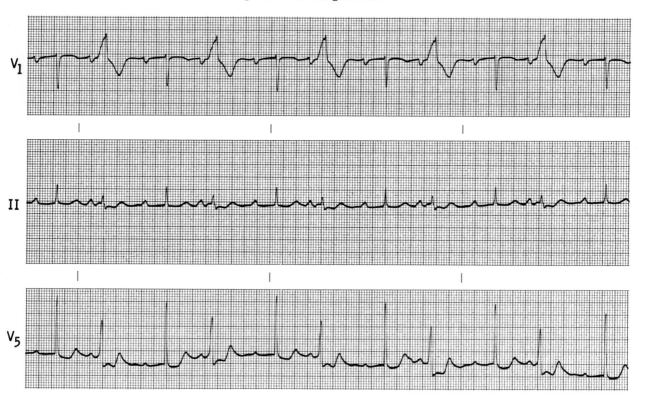

Case 130: Diagnosis

The underlying cardiac rhythm is sinus (rate: 72 beats per minute) with markedly prolonged P-R interval (0.36 second)—first degree A-V block. There are frequent VPCs causing ventricular septum, judging from their morphology—upright (positive) in both right and left precordial leads (see Case 79). As mentioned previously, the VPCs arising from the left ventricle and ventricular septum are commonly encountered in patients with organic heart disease and/or digitalis toxicity (see Cases 77 and 79). Conversely, right VPCs are common in apparently healthy individuals (see Case 78).

Ventricular bigeminy is considered to be a hallmark of digitalis toxicity by many physicians.

Left atrium is markedly enlarged, and left ventricular hypertrophy can be diagnosed without any difficulty.

Case 131

A 78-year-old woman with a long-standing congestive heart failure was admitted to the cardiac service because she developed a very slow heart rate associated with worsening of the cardiac condition. Digitalis toxicity was suspected.

1. *What is your cardiac rhythm diagnosis?*
2. *What is the best therapeutic approach?*

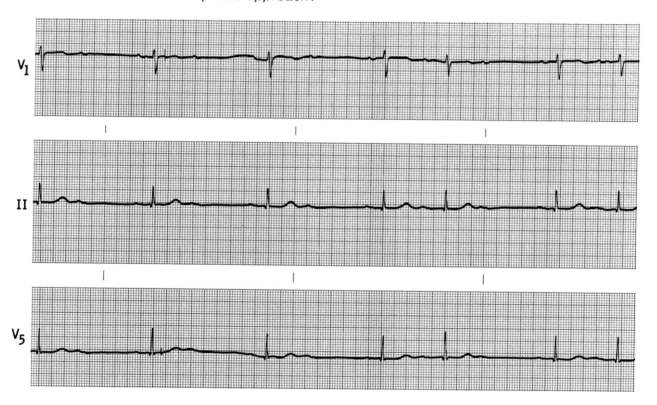

Case 131: Diagnosis

The cardiac rhythm is sinus (atrial rate: 68 beats per minute) with 3:2 Wenckebach A-V block and an area of 2:1 A-V block. During 2:1 A-V block, extremely slow ventricular rate (rate: 34 beats per minute) is produced. As described previously, 2:1 A-V block is usually a variant of Wenckebach A-V block when both arrhythmias occur periodically in the same ECG tracing. In general, 2:1 A-V block with normal QRS complexes is a variant of Wenckebach A-V block. The mechanism of Wenckebach A-V block has been described previously (see Case 37).

The first and the most important therapeutic approach to digitalis toxicity is, of course, immediate discontinuation of digitalis. If there are significant symptoms (e.g., dizziness, near-syncope, syncope, worsening of heart failure, etc.) and/or hemodynamic abnormalities (e.g., hypotension) directly due to slow heart rate, a temporary artificial pacemaker should be inserted.

Case 132

A 65-year-old woman with chronic congestive heart failure due to coronary artery disease associated with a long-standing atrial fibrillation (AF) developed a slow and regular heart rhythm, and the cardiac condition deteriorated progressively. Digitalis toxicity was suspected and she was admitted to the intermediate cardiac care unit.

1. *What is your cardiac rhythm diagnosis?*
2. *What is the other ECG abnormality?*
3. *What is the treatment of choice?*

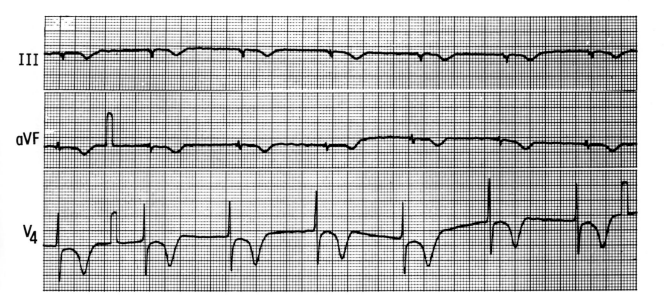

Case 132: Diagnosis

The underlying cardiac rhythm AF but the ventricular cycle is very regular. Thus, a complete rhythm diagnosis is AF with A-V junctional escape rhythm (ventricular rate: 53 beats per minute) due to complete A-V block producing complete A-V dissociation.

Diffuse myocardial ischemia is diagnosed because T waves are inverted in many leads (only 3 leads are shown here). In addition, diaphragmatic myocardial infarction (MI) is a strong possibility. By reviewing her past history, it was noted that she had suffered from diaphragmatic MI 3 months previously.

Needless to say, immediate discontinuation of digitalis is the first therapeutic approach. As long as the bradyarrhythmia does not cause significant symptom or hemodynamic abnormality, an artificial pacing is *not* indicated.

It should be noted that the incidence of digitalis toxicity increases in the presence of any active or acute heart disease (e.g., myocardial ischemia or infarction).

Case 133

This ECG tracing was taken on a 64-year-old woman with chronic congestive heart failure associated with a long-standing AF. Digitalis toxicity was suspected because her heart rate was progressively reduced associated with worsening of the cardiac condition.

1. *What is your cardiac rhythm diagnosis?*
2. *Is an artificial pacemaker indicated?*

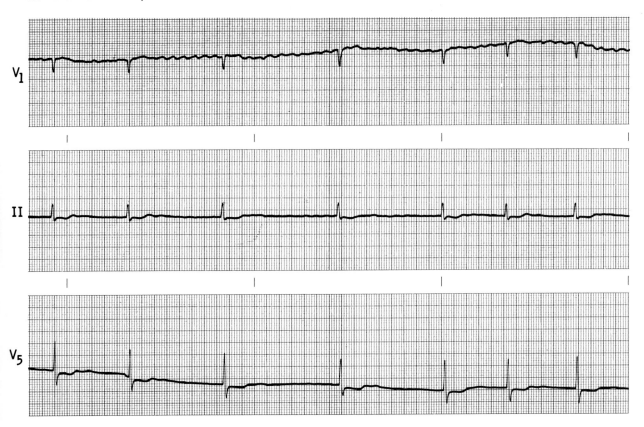

Case 133: Diagnosis

The underlying cardiac rhythm is atrial flutter-fibrillation, but the ventricular rate is very slow, yet irregular. Thus, the cardiac rhythm diagnosis of this tracing is atrial flutter-fibrillation with advanced A-V block causing a very slow and irregular ventricular cycle (ventricular rate: 34–55 beats per minute). The term, "atrial flutter-fibrillation" is used when the cardiac rhythm consists of a mixture of AF and atrial flutter— common occurrence.

Indication versus nonindication of a temporary artificial pacemaker will be determined primarily on the basis of the presence or absence of significant symptom and/or hemodynamic abnormality (e.g., dizziness, near-syncope, syncope, hypotension, etc.) directly due to slow heart rate. In most cases, discontinuation of digitalis is sufficient to treat digitalis-induced bradyarrhythmias.

Note prominent U waves compatible with hypokalemia. It has been repeatedly emphasized that hypokalemia predisposes to digitalis toxicity.

Case 134

These rhythm strips were obtained from a 59-year-old man with coronary heart disease and chronic AF. He was admitted to the hospital because of possible digitalis intoxication. Leads II-a and b and leads V_1-1 and b are continuous in each given lead.

What is the rhythm diagnosis?

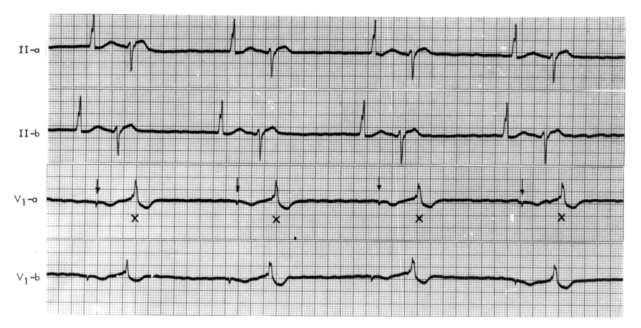

Case 134: Diagnosis

The underlying rhythm indicates AF, but there are two types of QRS complexes. The R-R intervals between QRS complexes indicated by arrows are regular, indicating independent ventricular activity. Thus, a final interpretation of this arrhythmia is AF with atrioventricular junctional escape rhythm (indicated by arrows) caused by complete A-V block, producing complete A-V dissociation and ventricular bigeminy (marked X).

This type of arrhythmia is an almost pathognomonic feature of digitalis intoxication.

Case 135

During digitalization, the cardiac rhythm is found to be regular in a 61-year-old man with chronic AF or flutter-fibrillation with congestive heart failure due to hypertensive heart disease.

1. *What is your cardiac rhythm diagnosis?*
2. *What is the most likely direct cause of this rhythm disorder?*
3. *What other ECG abnormality is present?*

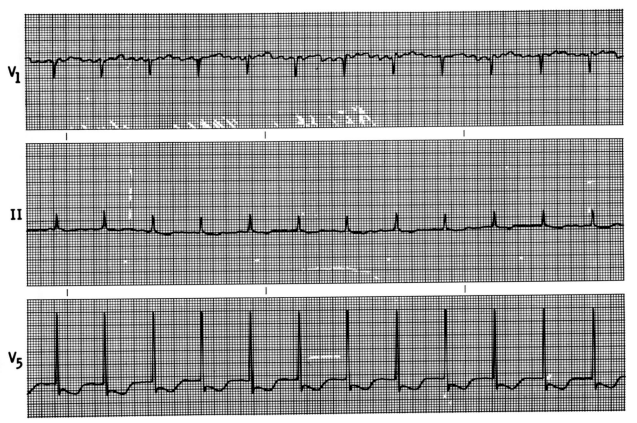

Case 135: Diagnosis

The underlying cardiac rhythm is atrial flutter-fibrillation, but the R-R interval is precisely regular. Thus, a complete cardiac rhythm diagnosis is atrial flutter-fibrillation with nonparoxysmal A-V junctional tachycardia (ventricular rate: 83 beats per minute) producing complete A-V dissociation.

In this case, nonparoxysmal A-V junctional tachycardia is responsible for the production of complete A-V dissociation. The cause for the genesis of nonparoxysmal A-V junctional tachycardia is, needless to say, digitalis intoxication. It should be re-emphasized that the most common cause of nonparoxysmal A-V junctional tachycardia is digitalis intoxication.

It is easy to recognize the evidence of left ventricular hypertrophy. In addition, coarse AF or atrial flutter-fibrillation often suggests left atrial hypertrophy.

Case 136

This ECG tracing was obtained from a 65-year-old man with hypertensive cardiovascular disease. Digitalis toxicity was suspected.

1. *What is your cardiac rhythm diagnosis?*
2. *What other ECG abnormality is present?*

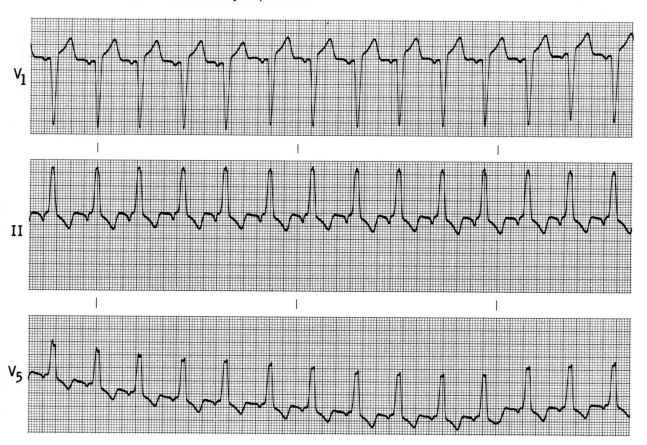

Case 136: Diagnosis

The cardiac rhythm diagnosis is nonparoxysmal A-V junctional tachycardia with a rate of 95 beats per minute. Note that each QRS complex is preceded by a retrograde P wave. In A-V junctional tachycardia, a retrograde P wave may precede or follow a QRS complex depending upon the timing of the atrial and ventricular activation. Obviously, the retrograde P wave precedes the QRS complex when the atrial activation takes place earlier than the ventricular activation, and vice versa. When the atrial and ventricular activation occurs simultaneously, the retrograde P wave will be superimposed on the QRS complex leading to absent P wave. Needless to say, no P wave is present in A-V junctional tachycardia when the underlying rhythm is AF atrial flutter.

Because of the pre-existing left bundle branch block (LBBB), ventricular tachycardia is superficially simulated. LBBB is very common in patients with hypertensive cardiovascular disease.

Case 137

Cardiology consultation was requested on a 65-year-old man with coronary heart disease because he developed a cardiac arrhythmia suddenly during digitalization.

1. *What is your cardiac rhythm diagnosis?*
2. *What other ECG abnormality is present?*

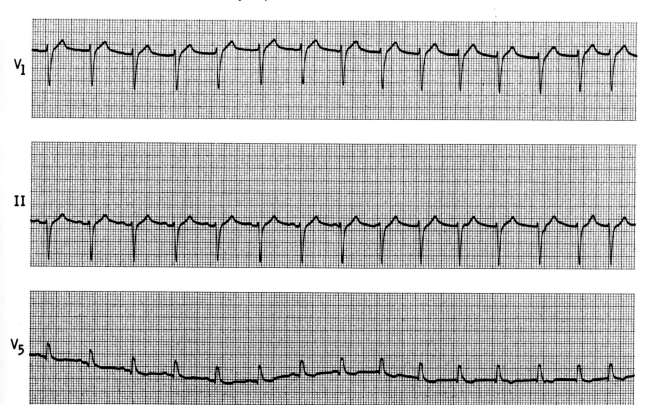

V₁

II

V₅

Case 137: Diagnosis

The underlying cardiac rhythm is sinus (rate: 92 beats per minute), but there is intermittent nonparoxysmal A-V junctional tachycardia (rate: 98 beats per minute) producing incomplete A-V dissociation (the last half of the tracing). Note a ventricular captured beat (the last beat of the tracing).

The diagnosis of left anterior hemiblock can be made on the basis of marked left axis deviation of the QRS complexes (the QRS axis is estimated to be −60 degrees). In addition, lateral MI can be diagnosed. The tall T wave in lead V_1 is suggestive of posterior myocardial ischemia.

Case 138

This ECG tracing was taken on a 59-year-old man with a previous heart attack 6 months earlier because digitalis toxicity was suspected. He has been taking digoxin 0.25 mg. once and hydrochlorothiazide 50 mg. twice daily for chronic congestive heart failure and mild hypertension.

1. *What is your cardiac rhythm diagnosis?*
2. *What other ECG abnormalities are present?*

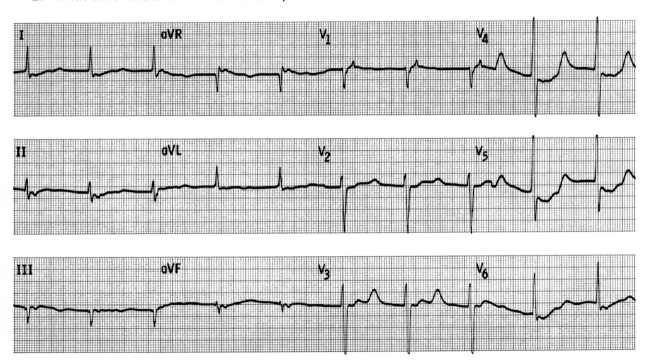

Case 138: Diagnosis

The cardiac rhythm is A-V junctional escape rhythm with a rate of 57 beats per minute. Note that each QRS complex is followed by a retrograde P wave. The status of the sinus node function is not exactly certain, but sinus arrest is a good possibility. In fact, sinus arrest is a common end result of advanced digitalis toxicity by virtue of the depressive action of the drug on the sinus node.

The striking ECG abnormality in this tracing is prominent U waves indicative of hypokalemia induced by diuretic therapy (hydrochlorothiazide). It is a well known fact that hypokalemia frequently predisposes to digitalis intoxication. Other ECG abnormalities include old diaphragmatic MI and left ventricular hypertrophy.

His serum digoxin level was reported to be 3.8 ng./ml., whereas the serum potassium value was 3.0 mEq./L.

Case 139

A 64-year-old hypertensive man with coronary artery disease was seen in the cardiac clinic because his cardiac rhythm had changed recently. Digitalis intoxication was suspected.

1. *What is your cardiac rhythm diagnosis?*
2. *What other ECG abnormalities are present?*

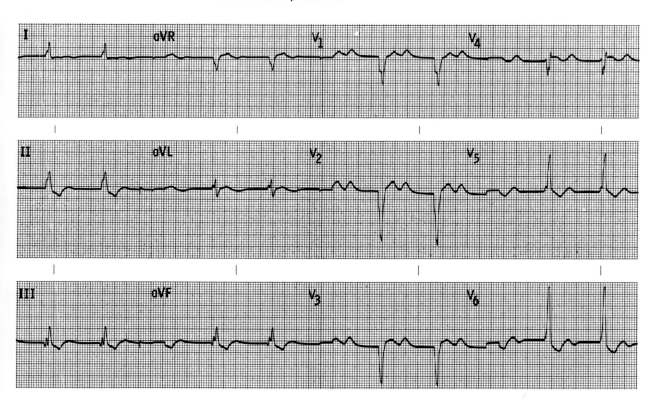

Case 139: Diagnosis

The cardiac rhythm is nonparoxysmal A-V junctional tachycardia with a rate of 67 beats per minute. Note retrograde P waves which follow QRS complexes. The QRS complex is broad as a result of the pre-existing LBBB.

Hypokalemia can be diagnosed without any difficulty on the basis of prominent U waves, particularly in leads V_{1-5}. Digitalis toxicity is easily produced when there is hypokalemia. In addition, old diaphragmatic MI is strongly suggested. As emphasized previously, LBBB is common in patients with hypertension, and hypertension is one of the major risk factors for coronary artery disease.

Case 140

This ECG tracing was obtained from a 56-year-old woman with long-standing rheumatic heart disease. She was admitted to the hospital because of increasing symptoms of heart failure in spite of maintenance digitalization and diuretic therapy.

1. *What is the rhythm diagnosis?*
2. *What is the most likely cause of this arrhythmia?*

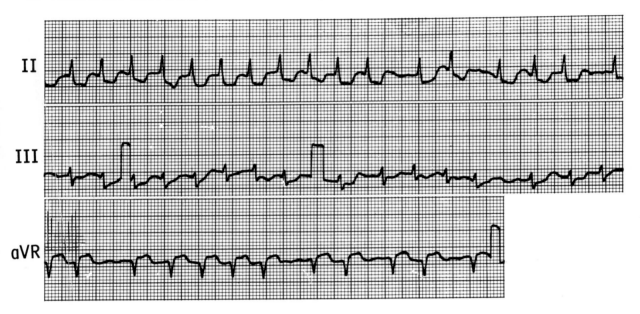

Case 140: Diagnosis

The basic rhythm indicates AF, but there are group beats followed by ventricular pauses. In addition, it should be noted that the R-R intervals progressively shorten until ventricular pause occurs in some areas. Thus, this tracing most likely represents AF and A-V junctional tachycardia with varying degree Wenckebach exit block producing A-V dissociation. Wenckebach A-V block has been described fully in Case 37.

A-V junctional tachycardia, especially in the presence of pre-existing AF, nearly always indicates digitalis intoxication.

Case 141

A 71-year-old woman with hypertensive cardiovascular disease was admitted to the intermediate cardiac care unit because of possible digitalis intoxication. Her cardiac rhythm had changed recently.

1. *What is your cardiac rhythm diagnosis?*
2. *What other ECG abnormality is present?*

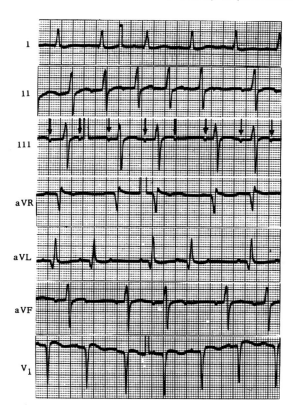

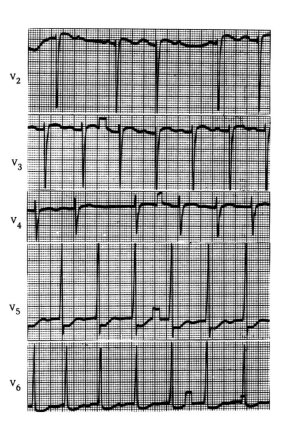

Case 141: Diagnosis

Arrows indicate P waves which are inverted in leads II, III, and aVF and upright in leads aVR and aVL. Thus, the atria are activated in a retrograde fashion. The complete rhythm diagnosis of this tracing is nonparoxysmal A-V junctional tachycardia (atrial rate: 115 beats per minute) with predominantly 3:2 Wenckebach A-V (forward or antegrade) block causing a regular irregularity of the ventricular cycle in most areas.

The diagnosis of severe left ventricular hypertrophy is obvious. Hypertension is the most common cause of left ventricular hypertrophy. Note that leads V_{3-6} are half-standardized.

Frequent occurrence of nonparoxysmal A-V junctional tachycardia in digitalis intoxication has been repeatedly emphasized.

Case 142

A temporary artificial pacemaker was inserted on a 54-year-old man with cardiomyopathy because of periodic occurrence of slow heart rhythm. Digitalis toxicity was suspected.

What is your cardiac rhythm diagnosis?

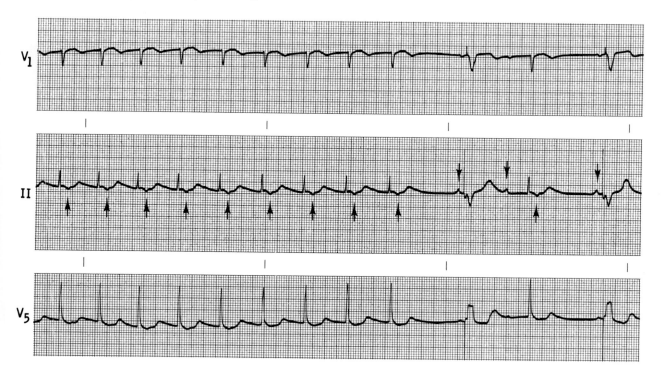

Case 142: Diagnosis

Downward arrows indicate sinus P waves, whereas upward arrows indicate retrograde P waves. Thus, it is easy to recognize that there are 2 kinds of P waves. The cardiac rhythm is sinus with marked first degree A-V block (P-R interval: 0.40 second) and intermittent reciprocating tachycardia (rate: 86 beats per minute—indicated by upward arrows). Note that a retrograde P wave (indicated by upward arrows) follows each QRS complex during a reciprocating tachycardia. It is a well known fact that reciprocating beats, rhythm, or tachycardia can be easily initiated when there is a significant depression in the A-V junction.

Note 2 pacemaker-induced ventricular beats. The pacing rate was set slower than the usual rate in this patient. The artificial pacemaker was unable to prevent the initiation of reciprocating tachycardia.

Case 143

This ECG tracing was obtained from a 63-year-old female with probable digitalis intoxication.

What is the ECG diagnosis?

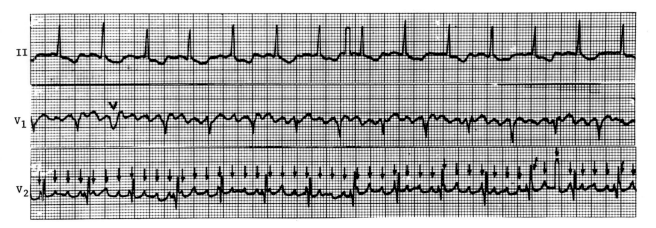

Case 143: Diagnosis

Arrows indicate atrial activities. The rhythm shows atrial flutter (atrial rate: 333 beats per minute) with nonparoxysmal A-V junctional tachycardia (ventricular rate: 100 beats per minute) producing complete atrioventricular dissociation. The rhythm superficially appears to be atrial flutter with 4:1 A-V block. However, it is obvious that atrial and ventricular activities are independent throughout. Note a VPC (marked V). Nonparoxysmal A-V junctional tachycardia during digitalis therapy almost always indicates digitalis intoxication, especially in the presence of pre-exisiting AF of atrial flutter.

Case 144

Both tracings (A and B) were obtained from the same patient on the same day only a few minutes apart. This patient had been taking 2 kinds of medication. Leads II-a, b, and c are continuous in both tracings.

1. *What is your cardiac rhythm diagnosis of both ECG tracings?*
2. *What medication(s) is (are) responsible for the production of these ECG abnormalities including a life-threatening arrhythmia?*

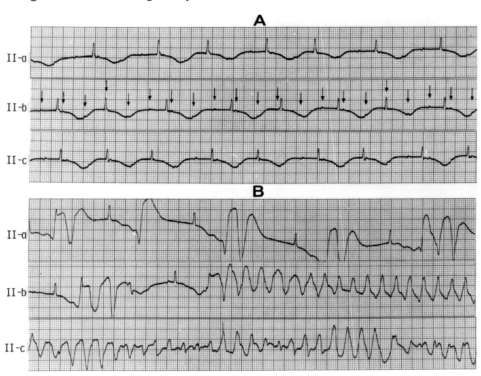

Case 144: Diagnosis

Tracing A: Arrows indicate ectopic P waves. The cardiac rhythm is atrial tachycardia (rate: 150 beats per minute—indicated by arrows) with varying Wenckebach A-V block. This cardiac arrhythmia is obviously due to digitalis toxicity (see Cases 61, 128, and 129). Another striking ECG abnormality is markedly prolonged Q-T interval with broad T wave due to quinidine. It has been well documented that serum digoxin level is often elevated when digoxin and quinidine are given together.

Tracing B: Within a few minutes, this patient developed multiformed ventricular tachycardia provoked by frequent VPCs with the R-on-T phenomenon leading to ventricular fibrillation. Again, markedly prolonged Q-T interval with broad T wave due to quinidine is responsible for the production of the R-on-T phenomenon. Thus, ventricular fibrillation is the end result of frequent VPCs (due to digitalis toxicity) with the R-on-T phenomenon due to the prolonged Q-T interval from quinidine. This type of irregular and multiformed ventricular tachycardia (prefibrillatory ventricular tachycardia) has been termed "torsades de pointes." Detailed descriptions regarding torsades de pointes are found elsewhere (see Case 185).

Case 145

A 70-year-old thin woman with a 6-year history of chronic renal failure of unknown etiology has been taking digoxin 0.125 mg. daily for chronic congestive heart failure. She underwent hemodialysis 3 times weekly. During dialysis she experienced sudden onset of palpitations and was found to have AF with a rapid ventricular response. Because of persisting rapid ventricular response in AF following additional digitalization (0.75 mg. of digoxin by mouth in 3 divided doses), elective cardioversion was attempted. Arrows indicate applications of direct current shock on 2 different occasions.

1. *What are the electrophysiologic events following direct current shocks?*
2. *What is (are) the fundamental mechanism(s) responsible for the production of new arrhythmias?*

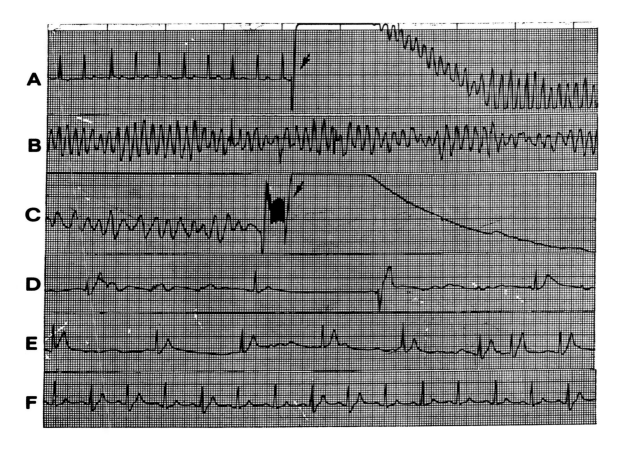

Case 145: Diagnosis

The rhythm (lead II) strips A-F are continuous. Arrows indicate applications of direct current (DC) shock. Ventricular fibrillation was provoked when DC shock, 50 ws. was applied (arrow in strip A), 400 w-sec. was effective to terminate the DC shock-induced ventricular fibrillation. Note a long period of ventricular standstill followed by unstable and slow ventricular and A-V junctional escape rhythms until sinus rhythm was restored (strips C-F). There is intermittent right bundle branch block during sinus rhythm, as evidenced in strip F.

There are 2 definite reasons why ventricular fibrillation was provoked in this patient. First of all, DC shock was applied during a vulnerable period of the ventricles (the R-on-T phenomenon) for the treatment of AF (arrow in strip A). The second reason is that the threshold of the initiation of ventricular fibrillation is markedly reduced during digitalization, particularly in patients with digitalis toxicity so that DC shock may easily provoke ventricular fibrillation under this circumstance. Thus, it can be said that DC shock is relatively contraindicated during digitalization. Fortunately, sinus rhythm is restored following the second DC shock. RBBB during sinus rhythm is an incidental finding.

Case 146

This ECG tracing was obtained from a 73-year-old man with chronic congestive heart failure. Digitalis toxicity was suspected initially because of frequent bizarre beats, but the diagnosis of digitalis toxicity was excluded later.

1. *What is your cardiac rhythm diagnosis?*
2. *What cardiac arrhythmias may be considered to be NOT digitalis-induced?*

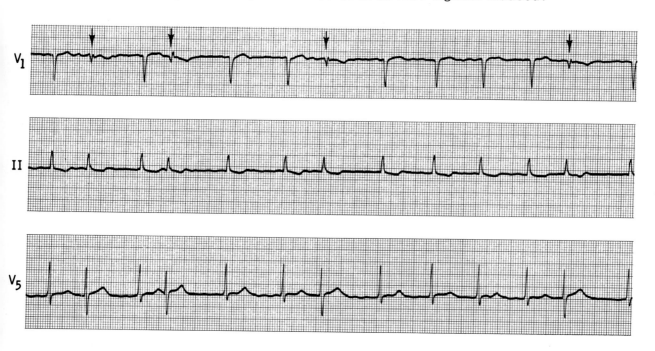

Case 146: Diagnosis

The underlying cardiac rhythm is AF, but there are frequent bizarre QRS complexes (indicated by arrows). At a glance, the bizarre beats appear to be frequent VPCs. However, the diagnosis of ventricular parasystole (rate: 47 beats per minute) can be entertained on the basis of varying coupling intervals (the *coupling interval* is defined as the interval from the ectopic beat to the preceding beat of the basic rhythm) with constant short interectopic intervals.

It has been shown that parasystole is not related to digitalis. The term, "nondigitalis-induced arrhythmias" is used to describe all cardiac arrhythmias which are *not* induced by digitalis. *Nondigitalis-induced arrhythmias* may include:

- Parasystole (atrial, A-V junctional, or ventricular)
- Mobitz type II A-V block
- Sinus tachycardia
- Paroxysmal A-V junctional tachycardia
- Intraventricular blocks (all types)

chapter 8

Arrhythmias Related to Artificial Pacemakers

Case 147

A permanent artificial pacemaker was implanted 6 years ago for the treatment of fainting episodes, and the pulse generator was replaced 3 years ago. Leads II-a, b, and c are not continuous.

1. *What is the mode of artificial pacing?*
2. *What is the underlying atrial mechanism?*
3. *What other arrhythmia is present?*

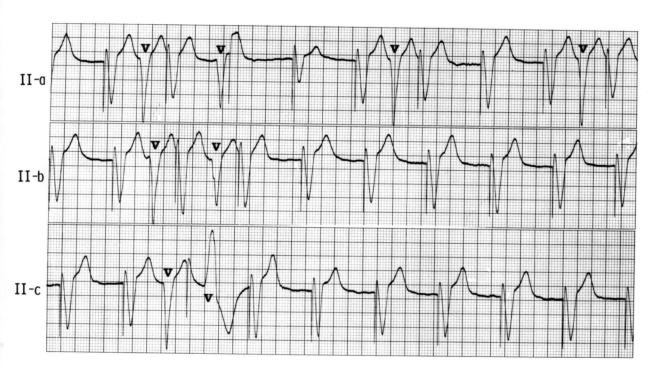

Case 147: Diagnosis

The mode of artificial cardiac pacing is, without doubt, fixed rate ventricular pacing with a rate of 70 beats per minute. It should be noted that the ventricular pacing spikes occur constantly regardless of the underlying cardiac rhythm—the characteristic feature of the fixed rate ventricular pacing mode.

The underlying atrial mechanism is atrial fibrillation and there are frequent multifocal ventricular premature contractures (VPCs) (marked V). Note that most VPCs are interpolated. When VPCs occur frequently in the presence of the fixed rate ventricular paced rhythm, a very rapid ventricular rate is produced, and the patient often feels palpitations. Some artificial pacemaker spikes fail to capture the ventricles immediately after VPCs because the ventricles are totally refractory during that time. In addition, an artificial pacing spike is superimposed on the top of the T wave of the preceding beat (the 3rd spike in lead II-C)—the R-on-T phenomenon. As indicated earlier, ventricular fibrillation may be easily provoked because of low ventricular fibrillation threshold during the vulnerable period (see Case 144).

At the present time, a fixed rate pacemaker is not popular because of the above-mentioned potential complications, and it is progressively being replaced by various newer pacemakers with demand pacing modes.

Case 148

A permanent pacemaker implantation was performed on a 71-year-old man with Adams-Stokes syndrome 6 months previously. He had been taking digoxin 0.25 mg. daily for chronic congestive heart failure even after artificial pacemaker implantation.

1. *What is your complete cardiac rhythm diagnosis?*
2. *What is the mode of artificial pacing?*
3. *Is this artificial pacemaker functioning normally?*
4. *What is a possible cause responsible for the production of extra heart beats?*

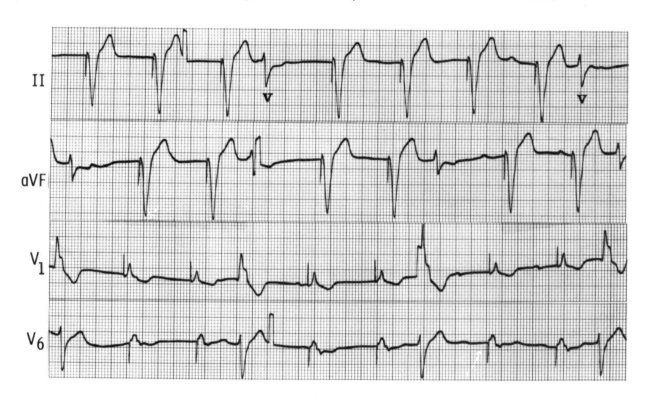

Case 148: Diagnosis

This ECG tracing reveals sinus bradycardia (atrial rate: 57 beats per minute) with a demand ventricular pacemaker rhythm (rate: 70 beats per minute) and frequent VPCs (marked V). The demand pacing mode is obvious in this tracing because the artificial pacemaker takes over the ventricular activity with the preset pacemaker escape interval following a VPC—the finding is in contrast to the fixed-rate pacing mode (see Case 147).

Malposition of the pacemaker electrode is suspected on the basis of upright (positive) QRS complexes of the paced beats in lead V_1. Remember that the QRS complex of the right ventricular paced beat should show negative (downward) QRS complex in lead V_1—the explanation comparable to the VPC arising from the right ventricle (see Case 78). In a broad sense, the malposition of the pacemaker electrode is a manifestation of the pacemaker malfunction, even though otherwise the pacemaker works normally. In fact, the malpositioned electrode as a result of a partial penetration into the septum had been corrected in this patient immediately.

Frequent VPCs were considered to be due to digitalis toxicity, and the drug was discontinued subsequently with further improvement of the cardiac condition.

Case 149

A temporary artificial pacemaker was inserted in a 64-year-old man with coronary artery disease. He was not taking any medication.

1. *What is the mode of artificial pacing?*
2. *What is the origin of the ectopic beats?*

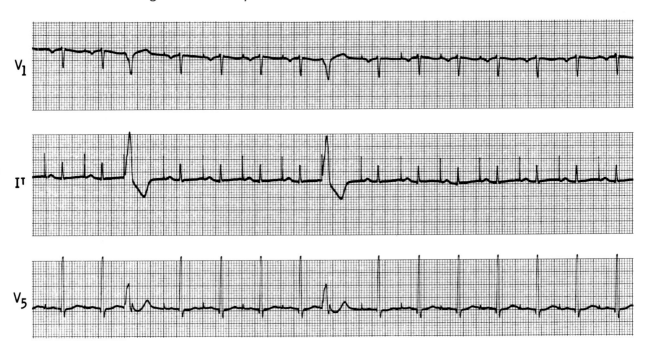

Case 149: Diagnosis

The underlying cardiac rhythm is right atrial pacemaker rhythm with a rate of 98 beats per minute. Note that every upright (positive) P wave in lead II is initiated by the artificial pacemaker spike and there is first degree A-V block (the P-R interval: 0.23 second).

There are frequent VPCs most likely originating from the right ventricle. The right VPC is diagnosed on the basis of a negative (downward) QRS complex in lead V_1 and upright (positive QRS complex in lead V_5, as far as the configuration of the ectopic beat is concerned (see Case 78).

Whenever VPCs occur, the expected pacing-induced P waves are not visible simply because the P waves are buried in the broad QRS complexes of the VPCs.

Case 150

An artificial pacemaker was implanted in a 37-year-old man with idiopathic cardiomyopathy associated with complete atrioventricular block. Leads II-a and b are not continuous.

What type of an artificial pacemaker was used in this patient?

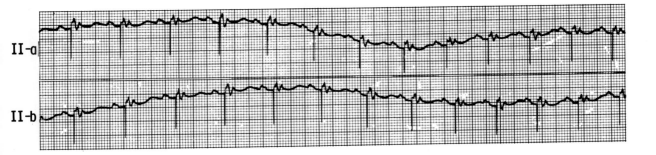

Case 150: Diagnosis

An atrial-synchronized artificial pacemaker (synchronized pacemaker, Nathan pacemaker, atrial triggered pacemaker) was used in this patient; it is a more physiologic type of artificial pacemaker than the asynchronous (ventricular) pacemaker.

In the atrial-synchronized pacemaker, the pulse generator is triggered by the natural P wave of atrial depolarization, and ventricular stimulation follows after an optimal delay corresponding to the P-R interval. In other words, an atrial-synchronized pacemaker functions as an electrical bundle of His. The major advantage of this type of pacemaker is its ability to provide maximum augmentation of the cardiac output at changing atrial rates in order to meet varying physiologic requirements. In addition, another benefit is the utilization of the atrial contribution to ventricular filling to further augment the cardiac output. Thus, the atrial-synchronized pacemaker is extremely valuable in younger or more active individuals. When atrial tachycardia or flutter occurs, the pacemaker induces A-V block of varying degrees, so that an optimum ventricular rate is maintained. On the other hand, when a marked slowing of the atrial rate or atrial asystole or electrical failure develops, a standby device automatically produces a ventricular rate of about 60 beats per minute as a ventricular fixed rate pacemaker.

An atrial-synchronized pacemaker is contraindicated in atrial fibrillation, marked sinus bradycardia, unstable atrial activity such as sino-atrial block or sinus arrest and atrial standstill.

Case 151

This ECG tracing was obtained from a 66-year-old woman with coronary artery disease. She was admitted to the cardiac care unit because of a recent heart attack.

1. *What is your cardiac rhythm diagnosis?*
2. *What ECG abnormality is present?*

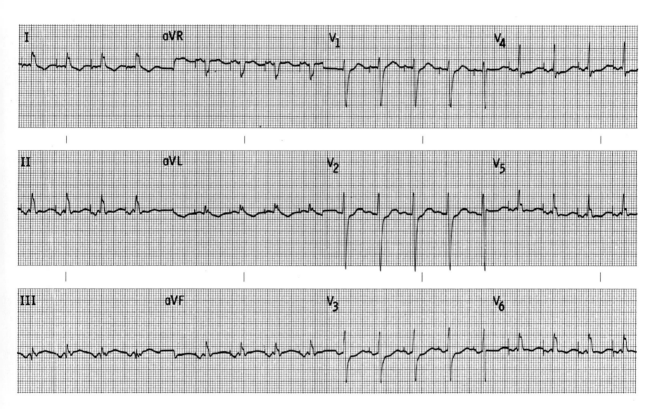

Case 151: Diagnosis

The cardiac rhythm diagnosis is coronary sinus pacemaker rhythm with a rate of 102 beats per minute. Note that each retrograde P wave is preceded by an artificial pacemaker spike with a constant P-R interval.

The diagnosis of diaphragmatic-lateral myocardial infarction (MI) can be made without any difficulty. The QRS complex is broad as a result of diffuse (nonspecific) intraventricular block—a rather common occurrence in patients with MI. Diffuse intraventricular block superficially resembles left bundle branch block (LBBB) (see Chapter 2).

This patient required a temporary pacemaker because of a transient but marked bradyarrhythmia.

This ECG tracing was taken on a 54-year-old man with coronary artery disease. He was not taking any medication.

What is your cardiac rhythm diagnosis?

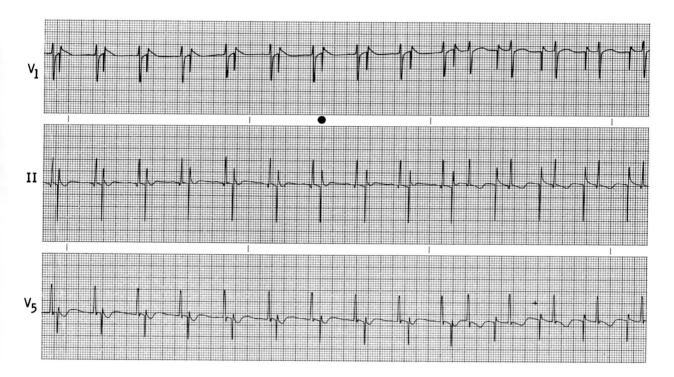

Case 152: Diagnosis

The underlying rhythm is normal sinus rhythm (rate: 84 beats per minute), but there is intermittent atrial (or coronary sinus) pacemaker rhythm with a rate of 83 beats per minute (the last 5 beats). Note that the artificial pacemaker spikes activate the P waves followed by constant P-R intervals and the QRS complexes in the last 5 beats. In the remaining portion of the tracing (the first two-thirds of the tracing), the sinus rhythm and the atrial pacemaker spikes (without activation of the heart) coexist independently with a very similar rate. During this portion of the tracing, an artificial pacemaker fails to activate the atria because of their refractory period.

Case 153

An artificial pacemaker was implanted on a 52-year-old man with coronary artery disease because of Adams-Stokes syndrome.

What is the mode of artificial pacing?

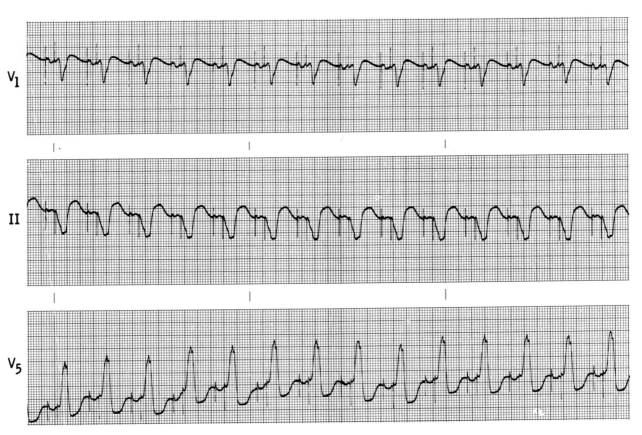

Case 153: Diagnosis

The cardiac rhythm is bifocal (A-V sequential) demand pacemaker rhythm with a rate of 94 beats per minute. Note that there are two sets of the artificial pacemaker spikes with constant intervals. In other words, one set of the pacemaker spikes activates the atria, whereas another set of the pacemaker spikes activate the ventricles sequentially with a constant preset P-R interval.

As far as the detailed features of the bifocal demand pacemaker are concerned, it consists of 2 demand units: a conventional QRS-inhibited ventricular pacemaker and a QRS-inhibited atrial pacemaker. In this model, the escape interval of the atrial pacemaker is designed to be shorter than that of the ventricular pacemaker. Thus, the difference between these two escape intervals is a determining factor for the A-V sequential delay. The bifocal demand pacemaker may be able to stimulate both atria and ventricles in sequence, whereas the unit may stimulate the atria alone or remain totally dormant, so that the pacemaker functions automatically according to the individual patient's needs.

In general, the bifocal demand pacemaker is considered to be indicated for a slow and unstable atrial mechanism associated with advanced or complete A-V block in that atrial contribution to the ventricular output is essential. Thus, the bifocal demand pacemaker is ideal for many patients with sick sinus syndrome (SSS), providing that the atrial mechanism is *not* atrial fibrillation or flutter (see Chapter 1).

Case 154

A permanent artificial pacemaker was implanted on a 37-year-old man with idiopathic cardio-myopathy in the treatment of complete A-V block.

1. *What is your cardiac rhythm diagnosis?*
2. *What is the mode of artificial pacing?*
3. *Is the artificial pacemaker functioning normally?*

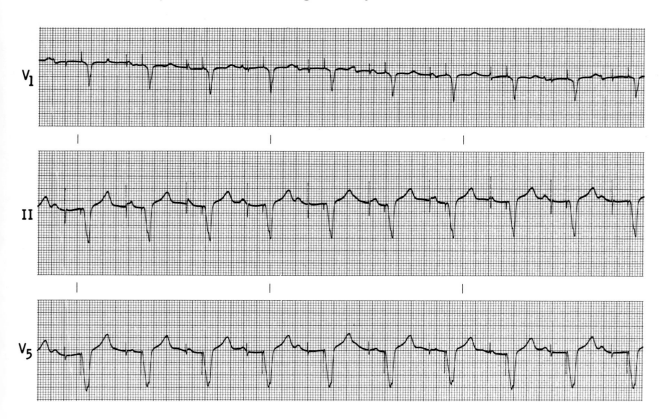

V₁

II

V₅

Case 154: Diagnosis

The cardiac rhythm diagnosis is sinus rhythm with an independent bifocal demand pacemaker rhythm (see Case 153). It is interesting to note that the atrial cycle is *not* regular, because the bifocal pacemaker activates both the atria and the ventricles sequentially (the 2nd, 3rd, 6th, 7th, and 8th beats) whenever the atria are not refractory. Otherwise, the bifocal pacemaker activates only ventricles while the atria are in their absolute refractory period as a result of the atrial activation by the sinus node. Thus, the first pacemaker spike fails to activate the atria in the remaining beats (the first, 4th, 5th, 9th and 10th beats). Since the sinus rate (the atrial rate of the sinus P waves: 72 beats per minute) is faster than the arltifical pacemaker preset rate (the pacing rate: 64 beats per minute), the atria are frequently activated by the sinus node. Of course, none of the sinus P waves are conducted to the ventricles. Remember that this patient required a permanent pacemaker for well established complete A-V block.

The bifocal demand pacemaker functions normally in this patient, but the benefit of the atrial contribution to improve the cardiac output is no longer present whenever the atria is activated by the sinus node prematurely. In a newer pacemaker with multiprogrammable capability, the pacing rate can be easily adjusted noninvasively according to the patient's needs. Accordingly, full benefits of the bifocal demand pacemaker can be accomplished in this patient when the pacing rate is increased above the sinus rate so that every pacing spike can activate the atria and the ventricles sequentially in order to provide the expected atrial contribution.

Case 155

This ECG tracing was obtained from a 44-year-old man with coronary and hypertensive heart disease. An artificial pacemaker was inserted because of intermittent and marked sinus bradyarrhythmia with advanced A-V block.

1. *What is your cardiac rhythm diagnosis?*
2. *What is the mode of artificial pacing?*
3. *Does the artificial pacemaker function normally?*

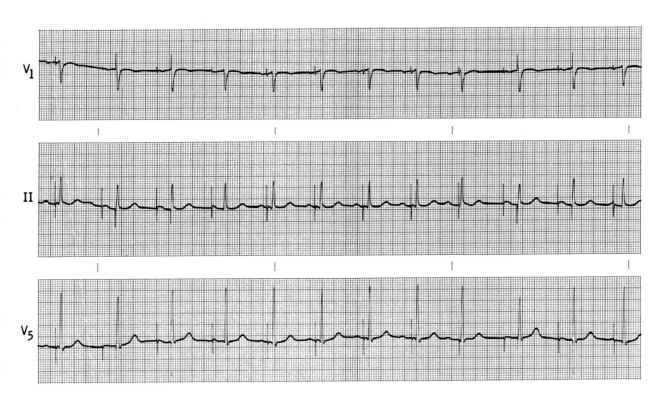

Case 155: Diagnosis

The underlying cardiac rhythm is sinus arrhythmia (atrial rate: 75 beats per minute) with first degree A-V block (P-R interval: 0.23 second). Whenever the sinus rate is reduced below the preset pacing rate, the artificial pacemaker activates the atria (the 2nd, 3rd, 10th, and 11th beats). In the remaining portion of the tracing, the atria are under the control of the sinus node. The ventricles are only occasionally partially activated by the artificial pacemaker following atrial activation sequentially (the 2nd, 3rd, 10th, and 11th beats).

The bifocal demand pacemaker is considered to function normally in this patient (see Case 153).

Case 156

These rhythm strips were obtained from a 74-year-old male who had had a permanent artificial pacemaker implanted for complete A-V block. Leads II-a, b, and c are continuous.

What is the ECG diagnosis?

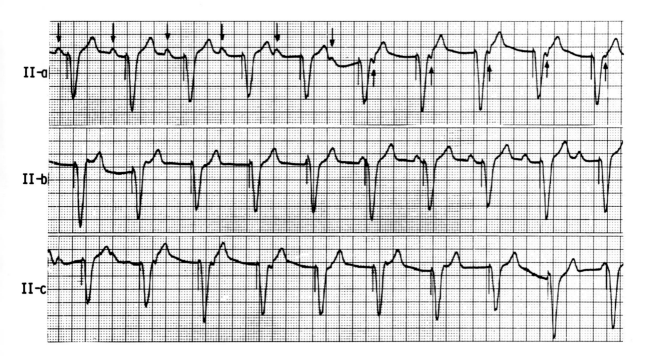

Case 156: Diagnosis

The rhythm is sinus (indicated by *downward arrows*) at a rate of 73 beats per minute with an artificial pacemaker-induced ventricular rhythm (rate: 68 beats per minute). It is interesting to note that there are frequent atrial captured beats (indicated by *upward arrows*). In other words, a retrograde ventriculoatrial conduction is intact in the presence of a complete antegrade A-V block. This finding is an obvious example of unidirectional block.

Case 157

A permanent artificial pacemaker implantation was carried out for a 49-year-old man with chronic complete A-V block.

1. *What is the cardiac rhythm diagnosis?*
2. *What is the atrial mechanism?*
3. *Is the artificial pacemaker functioning normally?*

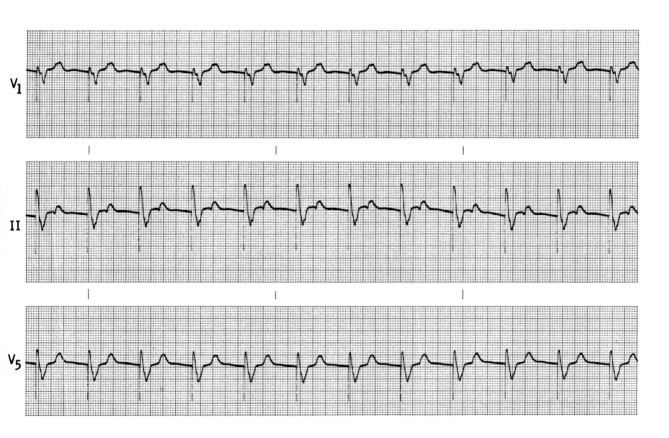

Case 157: Diagnosis

The cardiac rhythm is artificial pacemaker-induced ventricular rhythm with a rate of 72 beats per minute. It should be noted that every pacemaker-induced QRS complex is followed by a retrograde P wave—meaning atrial capture. In other words, the artificial pacemaker activates the ventricles and the atria sequentially. Thus, the atrial mechanism is consecutive atrial captured beats initiated by the artificial pacemaker. It is not uncommon that the retrograde ventriculoatrial conduction is perfectly intact in the presence complete forward (antegrade) A-V block as seen in this case. This electrophysiologic phenomenon is a good example to typify the unidirectional block.

The artificial pacemaker (demand ventricular pacing mode) functions normally.

Case 158

A permanent artificial pacemaker was implanted 2 years ago because of Adams-Stokes syndrome on a 66-year-old woman.

1. *What is your cardiac rhythm diagnosis?*
2. *Does an artificial pacemaker function normally?*

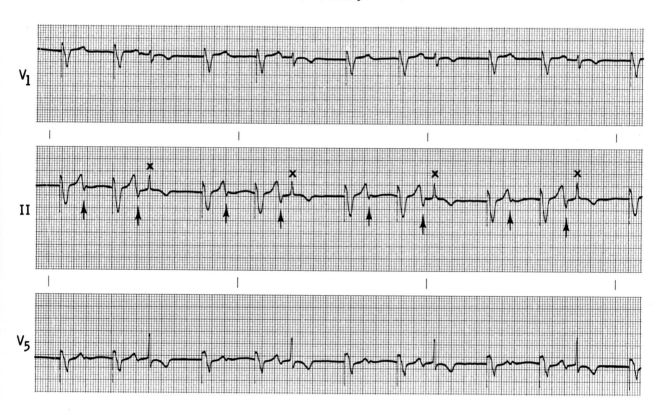

Case 158: Diagnosis

Arrows indicate retrograde P waves, and the P-P cycle reveals a regular irregularity. Namely, a short and a long P-P cycle alternate but the long P-P interval is shorter than 2 short P-P intervals. This ECG finding gives a clue for diagnosing Wenckebach phenomenon (see Case 37).

The cardiac rhythm diagnosis is an artificial pacemaker-induced ventricular rhythm (rate: 72 beats per minute) with Wenckebach ventriculoatrial block followed by a reciprocal beat (re-entrant beat or echo beat—marked X) occurring on every 3rd beat. It should be noted that the R-P intervals progressively lengthen until a reciprocal beat occurs.

Reciprocal beats, rhythm or tachycardia may easily develop in the presence of marked depression in the A-V junction leading to a longitudinal dissociation of the conductivity. When there is a marked prolongation of the retrograde ventriculoatrial conduction time (long R-P interval) in the presence of artificial pacemaker-induced ventricular rhythm, as seen in this case, a possibility of the production of reciprocal beats is very high. Once a reciprocal beat is produced under this circumstance, the re-entry cycle may repeat consecutively, leading to reciprocal rhythm or tachycardia.

The artificial pacemaker functions normally in this case as a demand ventricular pacing mode.

Case 159

A permanent pacemaker was implanted in a 63-year-old woman in the treatment of frequent syncopal or near-syncopal attacks. She was not taking any drug.

1. *What is the cardiac rhythm diagnosis?*
2. *What is the underlying cardiac disorder which required an artificial pacemaker?*
3. *What is the mode of artificial pacing?*

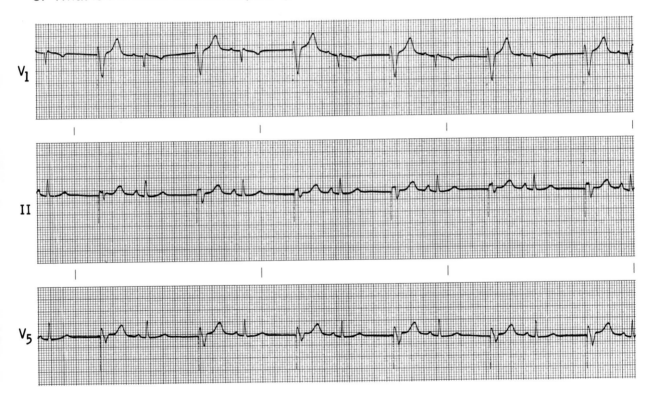

Case 159: Diagnosis

The cardiac rhythm is marked sinus bradycardia (atrial rate: 38 beats per minute) with an artificial pacemaker-induced ventricular beat which occurs on every other beat. Thus, the cardiac rhythm diagnosis is a form of "escape-bigeminy," and more specifically, "demand pacemaker escape-bigeminy."

The underlying cardiac disorder is obviously SSS, which is responsible for marked sinus bradycardia leading to frequent syncopal or near-syncopal attacks (see Chapter 1).

The artificial pacemaker functions normally with a preset rate of 72 beats per minute as a demand ventricular pacing mode.

Case 160

This ECG tracing was obtained from a 63-year-old woman who had received permanent pacemaker implantation 3 years previously because of frequent episodes of dizziness and near syncope. Her symptoms were abolished completely after pacemaker implantation.

1. *What is the cardiac rhythm diagnosis?*
2. *What is the underlying cardiac disorder which necessitated the artificial pacemaker?*
3. *What is the mode of artificial pacing?*

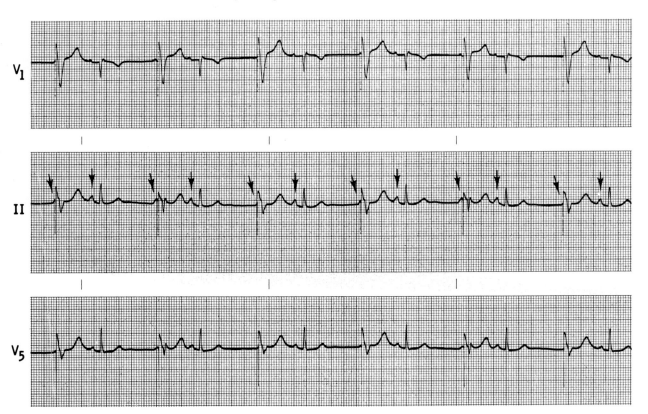

Case 160: Diagnosis

Arrows indicate sinus P waves, and the P-P cycle exhibits a regular irregularity. A long and a short P-P cycle alternate, but the long P-P cycle (interval) is shorter than 2 short P-P intervals. This regular irregularity of the P-P cycle represents 3:2 Wenckebach sino-atrial (S-A) block. Whenever the ventricular pause is longer than the preset pacemaker escape interval, the artificial pacemaker takes over the ventricular activity—the characteristic feature of a demand ventricular pacemaker. Again, the cardiac rhythm in this patient demonstrates "pacemaker escape-bigeminy" (see Case 159).

The underlying cardiac disorder in this patient is SSS, which produces 3:2 Wenckebach S-A block (see Chapter 1 and Case 1).

The artificial pacemaker functions normally in this case as a demand ventricular pacing mode.

Case 161

These cardiac rhythm strips were obtained from a 79-year-old man who had received a permanent artificial pacemaker 7 months previously.

What is your cardiac rhythm diagnosis?

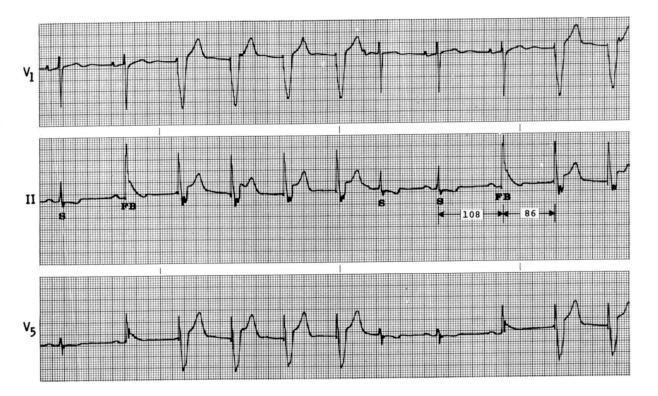

Case 161: Diagnosis

The tracing shows a ventricular demand pacemaker (Medtronic Model 5943)-induced ventricular rhythm (rate: 67 beats per minute) with intermittent sinus beats (marked S). Note that the pacemaker escape interval (1.08 seconds) is much longer than the consecutively occurring pacing intervals (0.86 second) because of *hysteresis*. There are occasional ventricular fusion beats (marked FB). (The numbers in this figure represent hundredths of a second.)

Hysteresis is a term which describes the difference between the rate at which a pacemaker initiates the pacing and the rate at which it discharges on a consecutive basis. The automatic interval is the time between 2 successive pacing spikes. The pacemaker escape interval is the length of the period from an intrinsic beat in the patient (sinus or ectopic) to the initial pacing impulse. An example of 10-beat hysteresis would be when a pacemaker does not fire until the patient's rate drops to 60 beats per minute or lower, at which time it starts pacing automatically at 70 beats per minute. This type of hysteresis is seen in the Medtronic Models 5943 and 5843 and the General Electric series A2075.

The only apparent advantage to hysteresis appears in its ability to preserve sinus rhythm. This is accomplished because the patient's own intrinsic rhythm can fall to lower levels (due to the longer escape interval) before asynchronous pacing is initiated. Thus, during rest or sleep when the intrinsic rate tends to be slow, the pacemaker with hysteresis would not fire asynchronously until the rate is reduced below 60 beats per minute.

There are several disadvantages to hysteresis which should be emphasized. That is, many physicians may misinterpret the hysteresis as a malfunctioning pacemaker because of the difference between the consecutive pacing intervals and the pacemaker escape interval.

Another disadvantage is related to the longer escape interval. After a sensed premature contraction, there is the production of a longer-than-usual postectopic pause which often leads to a longer ineffective ventricular cycle. This is especially true following a VPC.

The effect of hysteresis on battery life of the pacemaker is not yet clear. Although hysteresis does not appear to increase battery drain, the question of whether it increases battery life is unanswered. Part of the problem is due to the fact that the feature of hysteresis may be needed frequently by some patients, and others may never obtain benefit from it.

Case 162

This ECG tracing was obtained from a 64-year-old woman with a permanent artificial pacemaker. She was brought to the emergency room because of a rapid heart action.

1. *What is the ECG diagnosis?*
2. *Is the artificial pacemaker working normally?*
3. *What is the treatment of choice?*

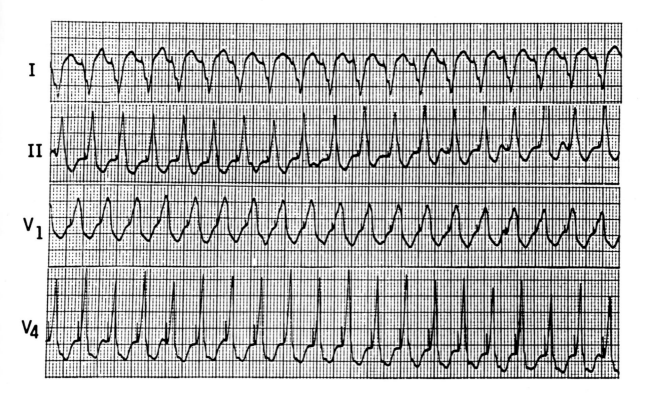

Case 162: Diagnosis

The cardiac rhythm is artificial pacemaker-induced ventricular tachycardia with a rate of 167 beats per minute as a manifestation of malfunctioning pacemaker. The preset pacing rate was 72 beats per minute.

Malfunction of an artificial pacemaker may occur with all commercially available models, but it is rare when dealing with newer models. The acceleration of the preset pacing rate is termed "runaway pacemaker," as seen in this case, and it is extremely rare today.

Malfunction of various artificial pacemakers may be manifested by:

(a) acceleration of pacing (runaway pacemaker)
(b) slowing of pacing (see Case 167)
(c) irregular pacing (see Case 167)
(d) failure of sensing and/or cardiac capture (see Cases 164 and 165) and
(e) combination of the above (see Cases 164, 166, and 167).

The runaway pacemaker is a medical emergency, and this type of tachycardia, needless to say, fails to respond to any antiarrhythmic agent. Thus, the treatment of choice is *immediate* discontinuation of the malfunctioning unit. This can be done by cutting the electrode wires near their attachments to the pacemaker. Connecting a temporary pacemaker to the bare electrode ends usually results in prompt recovery of most patients. A new, well functioning permanent unit should be implanted as soon as possible.

When the rate is extremely rapid in runaway pacemaker, the pacemaker stimuli are often insufficient to capture the ventricles, so that pre-existing A-V junctional or ventricular escape (idioventricular) rhythm as a result of complete atrioventricular block or any other bradyarrhythmias may reappear (see Cases 164 and 165).

Another abnormal finding in this tracing is the configuration of the QRS complex. That is, the QRS complex of the pacemaker-induced ventricular beat is upright (positive) in lead V_1—meaning malposition of the pacemaker electrode. Remember that the right ventricular paced beat should show a negative (downward) QRS complex in lead V_1.

Case 163

These cardiac rhythm strips were obtained from a 56-year-old woman with acute diaphragmatic MI. Artificial pacing with slightly overdriving rate (pacing rate: 90 beats per minute) was carried out in order to prevent recurrent drug-resistant ventricular tachycardias. The strips (monitor lead comparable to lead II) A to D are not continuous.

What is the cardiac rhythm diagnosis?

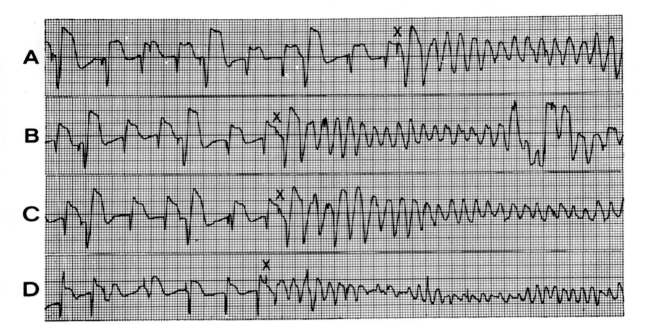

Case 163: Diagnosis

Ventricular fibrillation was provoked by the artificial pacemaker spikes with the R-on-T phenomenon (marked X). Fortunately, direct current shocks were successful to terminate the pacemaker-induced ventricular fibrillation in this case.

As has been repeatedly stressed (see Cases 106 and 144), the threshold for the initiation of ventricular fibrillation is significantly reduced during the vulnerable period of the ventricles corresponding to the duration of the T wave. Thus, ventricular fibrillation is easily provoked by any stimulus (e.g., VPC, artificial pacemaker spike, etc.) which is superimposed on the T wave of the preceding beat. In addition, the ventricular fibrillation threshold is further reduced when there is acute myocardial ischemia or MI, as seen in this patient. It should be noted that the danger of provoking ventricular fibrillation is always possible when one attempts to overdrive with an artificial pacemaker in order to suppress or to prevent any ectopic tachyarrhythmias.

Case 164

A 70-year-old woman was admitted to the intermediate cardiac care unit because of near-syncopal episodes associated with a very slow heart rate. An artificial pacemaker had been implanted 3 years previously for a persisting slow heart rhythm soon after a heart attack.

1. *What is your cardiac rhythm diagnosis?*
2. *Is an artificial pacemaker functioning normally?*
3. *What are the common causes of a failure of sensing and a failure of cardiac capture by the pacemaker?*
4. *What was the underlying cardiac disorder which required an artificial pacemaker?*

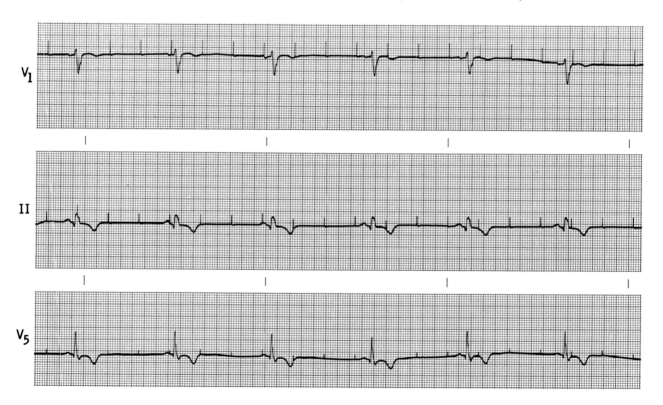

Case 164: Diagnosis

The cardiac rhythm is markedly slow sinus bradycardia (rate: 38 beats per minute), but there are regularly occurring artificial pacemaker spikes (rate: 120 beats per minute) without cardiac capture.

The artificial pacemaker is obviously malfunctioning, and it is manifested by acceleration of the pacing rate ("runaway pacemaker"), a failure of the cardiac capture and a failure of sensing.

Common causes of a failure of sensing and cardiac capture by an artificial pacemaker are summarized as follows:

Causes of Failure of Cardiac Capture

1. Pacemaker Malfunction (e.g. battery failure, electrode wire fracture, etc.).
2. Normally Functioning Pacemaker
   Poor electrode-endocardium contact (e.g., fibrosis, inflammation or edema in the region of the electrode)
   Advanced heart disease
   Electrolyte imbalance (hyperkalemia or hypokalemia)
   Drugs (procainamide, quinidine, propranolol, ?)
   Hypoxia, acidosis, or alkalosis

Causes of Loss of Sensing

1. Pacemaker Malfunction
2. Normally Functioning Pacemaker
   Low amplitude of intrinsic QRS complex
   Inappropriate intrinsic QRS vector perpendicular to pacemaker sensing axis
   Improper position of sensing electrode
   Electromagnetic interference
   Intrinsic QRS appearing in pacemaker refractory period
   Intraventricular conduction defects

This patient required a permanent pacemaker in the treatment of sick sinus syndrome (SSS) which was manifested by a persisting and drug-resistant symptomatic sinus bradycardia (see Chapter 1). SSS is not uncommon in patients with diaphragmatic MI, as seen in this case.

Case 165

Malfunction of an artificial pacemaker was suspected on a 51-year-old man. A permanent pacemaker with slightly overdriving pacing rate (80 per minute) was implanted about 4 years previously for SSS. He was not taking any drug.

1. *What is the underlying cardiac rhythm?*
2. *What is the manifestation of malfunctioning pacemaker?*

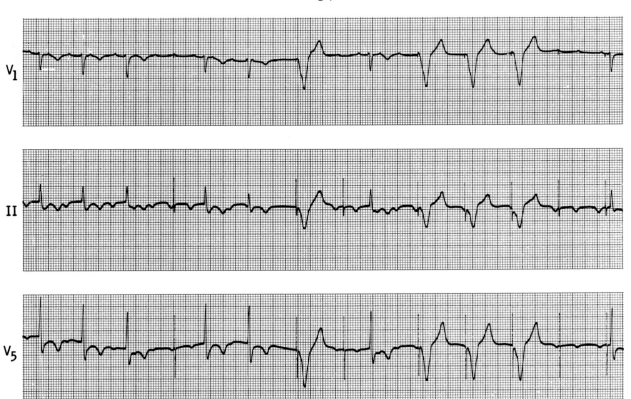

Case 165: Diagnosis

The underlying cardiac rhythm is atrial tachycardia (atrial rate: 170–190 beats per minute) with varying but advanced A-V block as a manifestation of SSS (see Chapter 1).

Malfunctioning pacemaker is manifested by intermittent failure of the ventricular capture. The malfunctioning pulse generator was replaced by a new unit.

Case 166

A 78-year-old man was admitted to the intermediate cardiac care unit for replacement of a malfunctioning artificial pacemaker. Initially, he was found to be in complete A-V block with a ventricular escape (idioventricular) rhythm of 35 beats per minute, and a permanent pacemaker was implanted. The preset pacing rate was 72 beats per minute.

What is the manifestation of malfunctioning pacemaker?

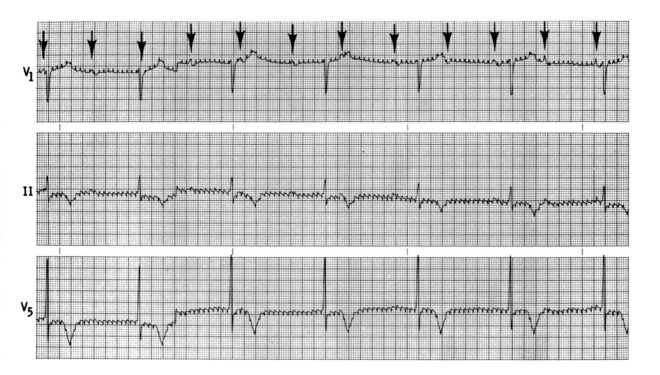

Case 166: Diagnosis

Arrows indicate sinus P waves. The tracing shows a far advanced runaway pacemaker with pacing rate of 750 beats per minute. None of the pacing spikes are followed by the QRS complexes. As a result, the pre-existing complete A-V block with slow ventricular escape rhythm (rate: 38 beats per minute) reappears. As a rule, a failure of cardiac capture almost always occurs when the pacing rate is accelerated markedly, as a manifestation of a malfunctioning pacemaker. The sinus P waves (indicated by arrows) are, of course, independent of the QRS complexes. Various manifestations of malfunctioning pacemaker have been described in detail previously (see Case 162).

Case 167

A permanent artificial pacemaker was implanted in an 83-year-old man for Adams-Stokes syndrome about 5 years ago, but he was not followed by a cardiac clinic or his physician on a regular basis. He was admitted to the cardiac service because a malfunctioning pacemaker was diagnosed.

1. *What is your complete cardiac rhythm diagnosis?*
2. *What is (are) the manifestation(s) of a malfunctioning pacemaker?*

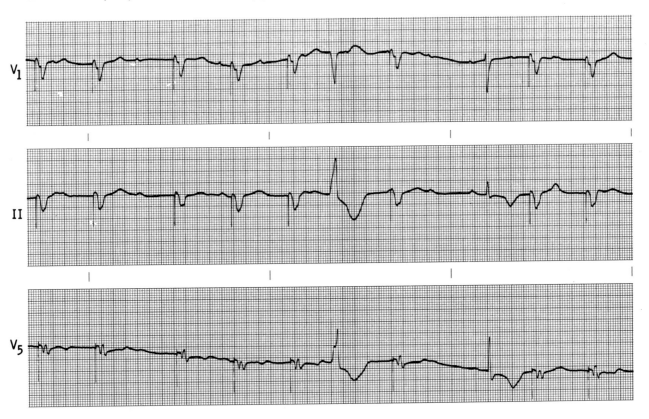

Case 167: Diagnosis

The underlying cardiac rhythm is sinus (atrial rate: 88 beats per minute) with advanced A-V block. The exact degree of A-V block can not be determined because an artificial pacemaker takes over the ventricular activity from time to time. The artificial pacemaker produces an irregular pacing cycle with occasional slowing. Thus, the malfunctioning pacemaker is manifested by an irregular and slow pacing.

Note a VPC (midportion of the tracing).

Case 168

A malfunctioning pacemaker was suspected on a 68-year-old woman who had received pacemaker implantation for SSS 1 year previously.

1. *What is your complete cardiac rhythm diagnosis?*
2. *What is a manifestation of malfunctioning pacemaker?*

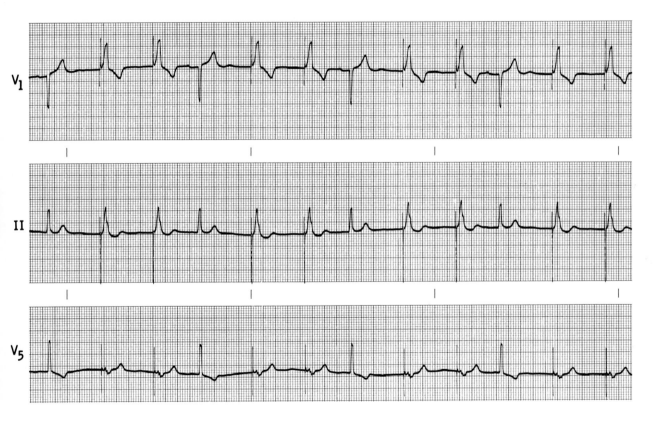

Case 168: Diagnosis

The underlying cardiac rhythm is mild sinus bradycardia with a rate of 50 beats per minute. An artificial pacemaker takes over the ventricular activity from time to time, leading to a regular irregularity of the cardiac cycle. Note normal sinus beats which occur on every third beat (the first, 4th, 7th, and 10th beats).

Malposition of the pacemaker electrode is diagnosed on the basis of the unexpected QRS morphology. Namely, the QRS complex of the paced beats shows upright (positive) configuration instead of the expected downward (negative) QRS complex in lead V_1 when considering the conventional right ventricular pacing. In a broad sense, the malposition of the pacemaker electrode is considered to be a manifestation of malfunctioning artificial pacemaker (see Case 162).

Case 169

A 65-year-old man who had had a permanent artificial pacemaker implanted 6 months previously was admitted to the hospital because of increasing symptoms of congestive heart failure in spite of maintenance digitalization. Leads II-a and b are continuous.

1. What is the rhythm diagnosis?
2. What is the most likely cause of this arrhythmia?

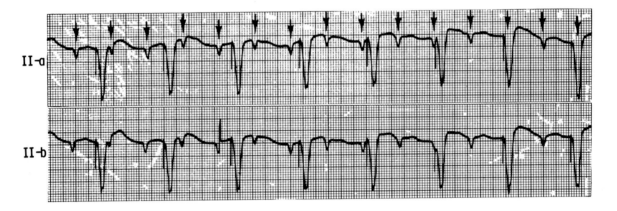

Case 169: Diagnosis

It is obvious that an artificial pacemaker-induced ventricular rhythm is present, and the pacing rate is found to be the same as the preset rate (57 beats per minute). It is interesting to note that all P waves are inverted in lead II (indicated by arrows), indicating retrograde conduction. Thus, the final diagnosis of this rhythm is nonparoxysmal A-V junctional tachycardia (rate: 105 beats per minute) in the presence of an artificial pacemaker-induced ventricular rhythm.

Digitalis intoxication was suspected, and digitalis was discontinued. Within several days, the sinus P waves returned. It is extremely important to recognize A-V junctional tachycardia in the presence of an artificial pacemaker-induced ventricular rhythm. Otherwise, digitalis intoxication may easily go unrecognized. Frequent occurrence of digitalis-induced nonparoxysmal A-V junctional tachycardia has been repeatedly emphasized (see Chapter 7).

Case 170

A 62-year-old man developed repetitive episodes of ventricular tachycardia and fibrillation, complicating acute MI. The ventricular tachyarrhythmias became refractory to various antiarrhythmic agents and direct current shock.

1. *What procedure was performed for the refractory tachyarrhythmias?*
2. *What is the rhythm diagnosis?*

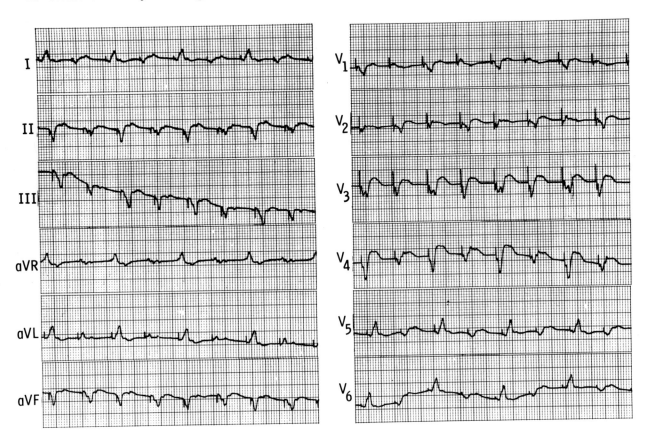

Case 170: Diagnosis

A temporary transvenous artificial pacemaker was inserted to the right ventricle in order to suppress ventricular tachycardia and fibrillation. The pacing rate (overdriving) was 115 beats per minute. It is a well known fact that any pacemaker (either sinus or ectopic) activity may be suppressed by another pacemaker if the latter produces impulses rapidly and actively. Once a pacemaker is suppressed by another pacemaker, the pacemaking function may not return for a long period of time. This electrophysiologic phenomenon is termed "postdrive inhibition phenomenon," which is often utilized to treat refractory tachyarrhythmias with the use of an artificial pacemaker.

Following insertion of an electrode catheter, the artificial pacemaker impulses capture ventricles as well as atria (note retrograde P waves following QRS complexes). In addition, the QRS configurations alter on every other beat, indicating 2:1 ventricular electrical alternans (see Case 178) in artificial pacemaker-induced ventricular rhythm. (Reproduced from E. K. Chung. *Principles of Cardiac Arrhythmias*, 2nd Edition. Baltimore, Williams & Wilkins, 1977; courtesy of Dr. Irving L. Rosen.)

Case 171

Coronary sinus pacing with overdriving rate (pacing rate: 90 beats per minute) was performed on a 58-year-old man with recent anterior MI in order to suppress and prevent recurrent and drug-resistant ventricular tachycardia and fibrillation. He also gave a history of previous diaphragmatic MI one year previously. The antiarrhythmic medications before the pacing included procainamide (Pronestyl) 750 mg. every 4 hours, quinidine sulfate 400 mg. every 6 hours, lidocaine 3 mg./minute and propranolol (Inderal) 1 mg. intravenously hourly. With the addition of overdriving pacing from the coronary sinus at 90 beats per minute, there was a decrease in the frequency of ventricular arrhythmias. The cardiac rhythm strips A, B, and C are continuous, and they represent lead II.

What is your cardiac rhythm diagnosis?

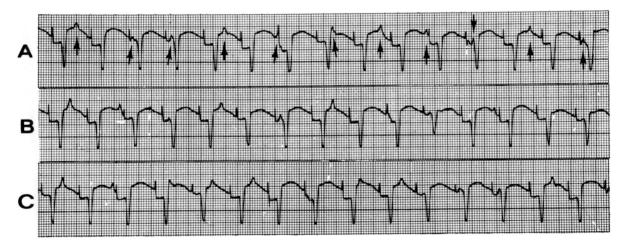

Case 171: Diagnosis

Arrows indicate P waves. These ECG rhythm strips demonstrate coronary sinus pacemaker rhythm (rate: 90 beats per minute) with an independent, unilateral atrial mechanism (indicated by arrows; atrial rate: 65–78 beats per minute) causing atrial dissociation. Note that none of the P waves are conducted to the ventricles.

Atrial dissociation is characterized by the presence of a unilateral atrial rhythm independent of the basic rhythm. There is no ventricular capture from the unilateral atrial focus regardless of the state of refractoriness of the ventricle or A-V junction In this way, it can be differentiated from atrial parasystole (see Case 174).

The most common form of atrial dissociation is a slow ectopic atrial rhythm with underlying sinus rhythm (see Case 183). Other unilateral foci have also been described including atrial tachycardia, atrial flutter, atrial fibrillation, and even unilateral sinus rhythm.

The present case represents atrial dissociation in which an artificial coronary sinus pacemaker rhythm is the basic mechanism, and the unilateral atrial rhythm is most likely originating from the sinus node.

The finding of the unilateral atrial mechanism with an underlying coronary sinus pacemaker rhythm is consistent with the previously proposed mechanism of protective entrance and exit blocks, causing electrical dissociation of a part of the right atrium. That is, the atrial pacemaker (possibly sinus node) was able to control only part of the right atrium and this area was protected from interference by the artificial pacemaker.

Case 172

Cardiology consultation was requested because of possible malfunction of an artificial pacemaker.

1. *What is your cardiac rhythm diagnosis?*
2. *What is the mechanism of this bigeminal rhythm?*
3. *Is an artificial pacemaker functioning normally?*

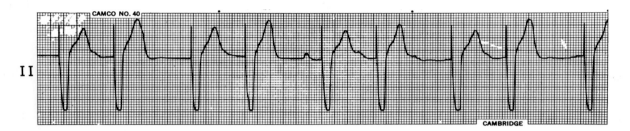

II

Case 172: Diagnosis

The rhythm strip exhibits an artificial pacemaker-induced ventricular rhythm with a regular irregularity of the pacing cycle, leading to a form of bigeminal rhythm. At glance, this cardiac arrhythmia appears to be a manifestation of malfunctioning artificial pacemaker, in view of possible improper sensing mechanism. However, it becomes obvious that the pacemaker is sensed by the T wave of the preceding beat on every other beat because the T wave is taller on every other beat due to 2:1 electrical alternans (see Case 178) involving only T waves. Therefore, this ECG finding is *not* a manifestation of malfunction.

This unusual pacemaker-induced bigeminal rhythm is an extremely rare occurrence, and it may be termed "artificial pacemaker bigeminy," which is a *pseudo*-malfunction of an artificial pacemaker.

chapter 9

Uncommon Cardiac Arrhythmias

Case 173

A 69-year-old man with a history of a heart attack 6 months previously was seen at the cardiac clinic for the evaluation of frequent ectopic beats. He was not taking any medication.

1. *What is your cardiac rhythm diagnosis?*
2. *What is the proper therapeutic approach?*

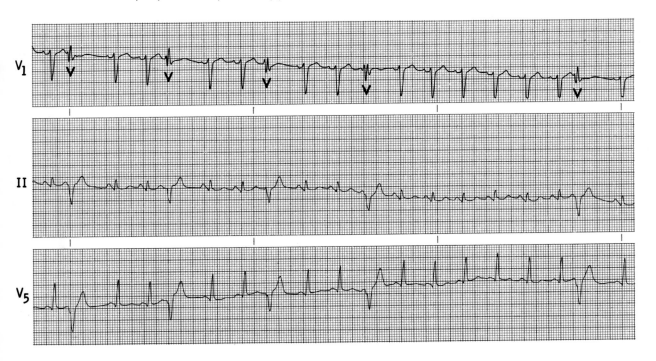

Case 173: Diagnosis

The underlying cardiac rhythm is sinus tachycardia with a rate of 113 beats per minute. There are frequent ventricular ectopic beats (marked V) which superficially appear to be ventricular premature contractions (VPCs). By a close observation, however, the diagnosis of ventricular parasystole (rate: 38 beats per minute) can be made on the basis of varying coupling intervals (the *coupling interval* is the interval from an ectopic beat to the preceding beat of the basic rhythm) with constant shortest interectopic intervals (the *interectopic interval* means the interval between two ectopic beats); namely, parasystole is an independent cardiac rhythm to the basic rhythm. When there is an exit block (an *exit block* means a block around the ectopic beat), the expected parasystolic impulse is not conducted to the heart, so that a long interectopic interval will be produced. Thus, a long interectopic interval shows multiples of the shortest interectopic interval. Since parasystole is an independent rhythm to the basic rhythm, fusion beats frequently occur (a *fusion beat* means that a cardiac chamber is activated by two or more different foci simultaneously leading to a mixed beat).

As far as the incidence of parasystole is concerned, this arrhythmia is found in 0.1–0.2% of the general hospital population. Ventricular parasystole is the most common parasystolic rhythm, and atrial or A-V junctional parasystole (see Cases 174 and 175) is encountered only occasionally in our practice. The usual rate of parasystole regardless of its origin is relatively slow—ranging from 30 to 60 beats per minute (Cases 173–175). On rare occasions, parasystole may produce tachycardia (see Case 176).

As far as the clinical significance is concerned, parasystole is more commonly found in cardiac patients than in healthy individuals, but the arrhythmia is usually benign and self-limited. Therefore, no treatment is indicated unless the individual complains of any symptom (e.g., palpitations, strange sensation in the chest, etc.) directly due to parasystole. One of the interesting observations is that parasystole has a tendency to be refractory to various antiarrhythmic agents. Another important clinical significance is that parasystole is *not* a digitalis-induced arrhythmia (see Chapter 7). Thus, the correct diagnosis of parasystole is essential, and otherwise, the arrhythmia may be misinterpreted as digitalis-induced VPCs during digitalization.

Case 174

This ECG tracing was taken on a 59-year-old woman with no demonstrable heart disease as a part of her annual medical check-up.

What is your cardiac rhythm diagnosis?

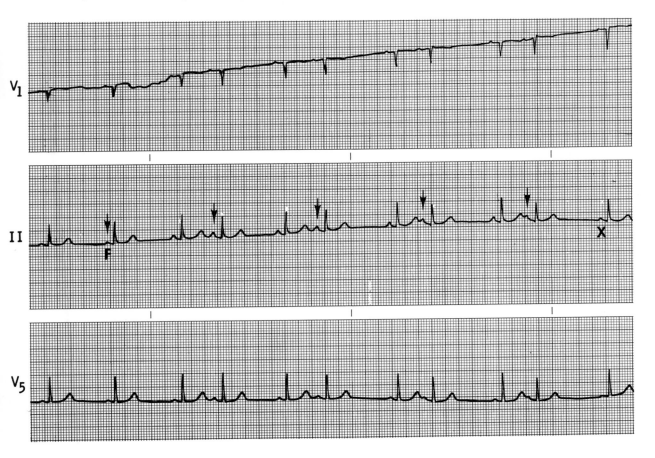

Case 174: Diagnosis

The underlying cardiac rhythm is sinus with a rate of 60 beats per minute. There are frequent atrial ectopic beats (indicated by arrows) which closely resemble atrial premature contractions (APCs). However, atrial parasystole can be diagnosed on the basis of varying coupling intervals and constant shortest interectopic intervals. The atrial parasystolic rate is 38 beats per minute. Note an atrial fusion beat (marked F). An atrial fusion is produced as a result of simultaneous activation of the atria by the sinus node and the parasystolic atrial focus.

It is interesting to note that one sinus P wave (marked X) immediately following the last parasystolic beat shows different configuration to compare with the remaining sinus P waves. This finding is termed "aberrant atrial conduction" or "Chung's phenomenon," which was described for the first time by this author more than 10 years ago. Chung's phenomenon may be observed following an APC (see Case 184) or atrial parasystolic beat. On rare occasions, Chung's phenomenon may occur following a retrograde P wave originating from a VPC or even ventricular parasystolic beat. Chung's phenomenon seems to be more commonly observed following a blocked APC or a retrograde P wave.

Detailed descriptions of parasystole are found elsewhere (see Case 173).

Case 175

Frequent ectopic beats were found on a 58-year-old apparently healthy man during a routine medical examination. He was totally asymptomatic.

What is your cardiac rhythm diagnosis?

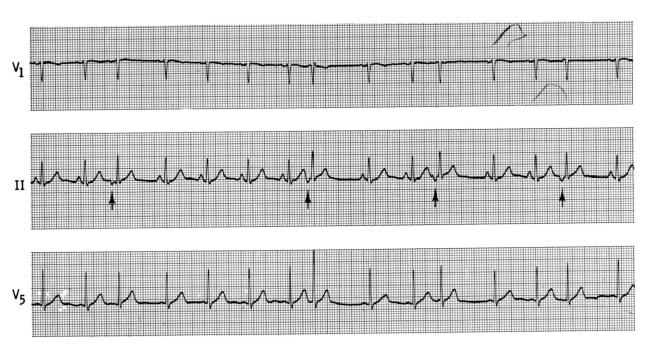

Case 175: Diagnosis

The underlying cardiac rhythm is sinus with a rate of 90 beats per minute. There are frequent A-V junctional beats (indicated by arrows) which superficially mimic A-V junctional premature contractions. Note that all ectopic P waves are conducted in a retrograde fashion (indicated by arrows), and each QRS complex is preceded by a retrograde P wave.

It is easy to recognize that the coupling intervals vary considerably. Yet, the direct parasystolic cycle cannot be found readily as a result of varying degree (3:1 and 4:1) exit block. Remember that the exit block is diagnosed when the expected ectopic beat fails to appear on the electrocardiogram because of a block surrounding the ectopic focus. It should be noted that some ectopic beats demonstrate a slightly bizarre QRS complex due to aberrant ventricular conduction (e.g., the 2nd parasystolic beat).

A complete diagnosis of this ECG tracing is sinus rhythm and A-V junctional parasystole (rate: 57 beats per minute) with varying degree exit block and occasional aberrant ventricular conduction. No treatment is indicated.

Case 176

A 38-year-old physician was referred to a cardiologist for evaluation of an arrhythmia associated with occasional palpitation. Leads II-a, b, c, d, and e are continuous.

What is the ECG diagnosis?

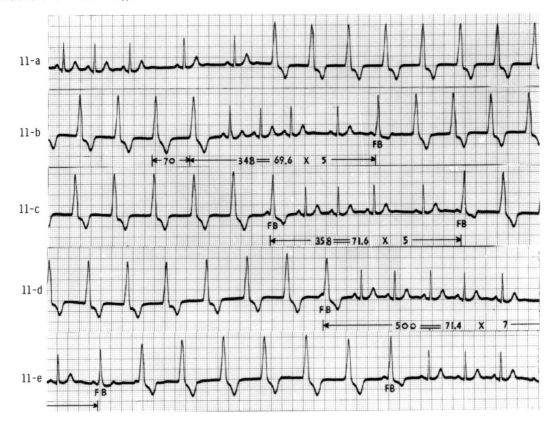

Case 176: Diagnosis

The tracing shows predominantly ventricular parasystolic tachycardia at a rate of 83 beats per minute and intermittent sinus rhythm at a rate of 93 beats per minute. Ventricular parasystole is diagnosed because the long interectopic intervals are multiples of the shortest interectopic interval. There are occasional ventricular fusion beats (marked FB). Ventricular tachycardia produced by a parasystolic mechanism often has a slower ventricular rate than ordinary ventricular tachycardia. A detailed description of parasystole is given in Case 173. (Numbers in this tracing represent hundredths of a second.)

Ventricular parasystolic tachycardia is usually benign and self-limited.

Case 177

This ECG tracing was obtained from a 59-year-old woman with no demonstrable heart disease.

1. *What is your cardiac rhythm diagnosis?*
2. *What is the clinical significance of this arrhythmia?*

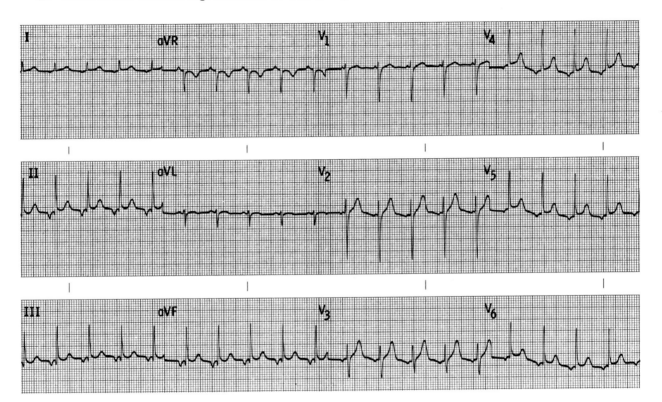

Case 177: Diagnosis

The cardiac rhythm is left atrial tachycardia with a rate of 110 beats per minute. The ectopic P waves are inverted in leads I, II, III, and aVF and V_{3-6} and upright in leads aVR, aVL, and V_1. The axis of the P waves is calculated to be −105 degrees.

Left atrial rhythm or tachycardia closely simulates A-V junctional rhythm or tachycardia because the ectopic P waves are conducted in a retrograde fashion in both conditions. The major important findings to support the diagnosis of left atrial rhythm or tachycardia and to exclude the diagnosis of A-V junctional rhythm or tachycardia consist of upright (positive) P wave without any negative component in lead V_1 with inverted (negative) P waves in leads I and V_{4-6}.

The clinical significance of left atrial rhythm or tachycardia is not clearly understood as of this writing. This arrhythmia has been encountered in healthy individuals as well as in patients with various cardiac conditions. No treatment is indicated for left atrial rhythm or tachycardia.

Case 178

This ECG tracing was taken on a 50-year-old woman with severe dyspnea and rapid heart action.

1. *What is your ECG diagnosis?*
2. *What is the most likely underlying disorder responsible for the production of this ECG abnormality?*

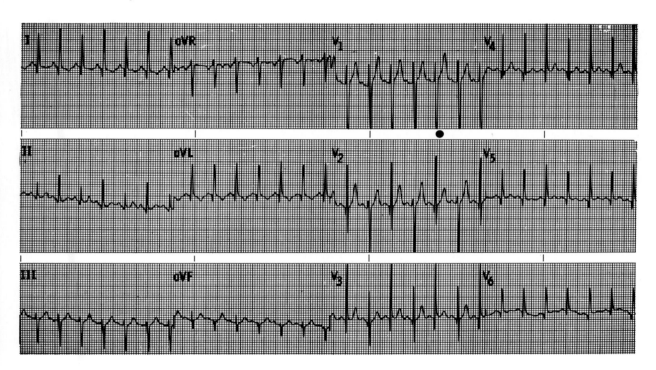

Case 178: Diagnosis

The cardiac rhythm is marked sinus tachycardia with a rate of 150 beats per minute. The configuration of the QRS complexes alters on every other beat—a finding termed 2:1 ventricular electrical alternans.

The electrical alternans is most commonly found in patients with massive pericardial effusion and less commonly in advanced congestive heart failure due to various underlying cardiac disorders. In every case of electrical alternans regardless of the underlying disease, the prognosis is generally grave. This patient was found to have a massive hemorrhagic pericardial effusion resulting from carcinomatosis originating from a breast cancer.

The electrical alternans most commonly involves the QRS complexes alone—termed ventricular electrical alternans as seen in this case. Less commonly, electrical alternans involves the P waves alone—called atrial electrical alternans. The term total electrical alternans is used when both the P waves and the QRS complexes are involved together. On rare occasions, electrical alternans may involve only S-T segment and/or T waves (see Case 172). The most common alternating ratio is 2:1 and other alternating ratios (e.g., 3:1 or 4:1) are very rare. The 2:1 electrical alternans during rapid ventricular pacing has been described previously (see Case 170).

The mechanism for the production of electrical alternans has not been fully understood, but an alternating refractory period of an involved portion of the heart is considered to be a major cause of this rare ECG abnormality.

Case 179

A 28-year-old pregnant woman with known rheumatic mitral stenosis, who had been taking digoxin (0.25 mg.) and hydrochlorothiazide (50 mg.) daily for 2 years, was admitted to the hospital because of increasing shortness of breath and ankle swelling over the previous 2 weeks. This ECG tracing was taken on admission. Leads II-a, b, and c are continuous.

1. *What is the rhythm diagnosis?*
2. *What is the most likely cause of this arrhythmia?*

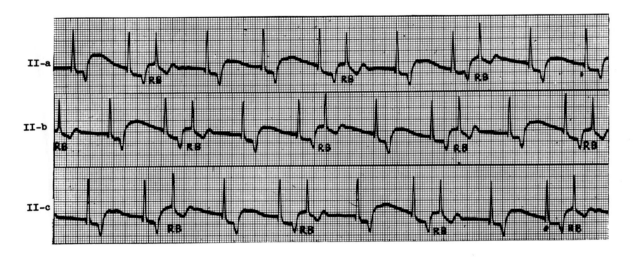

Case 179: Diagnosis

This tracing shows nonparoxysmal A-V junctional tachycardia (rate: 63 beats per minute) with Wenckebach retrograde ventriculoatrial block and frequent reciprocal beats occurring every third beat (marked RB).

A reciprocal beat is diagnosed when a retrograde P wave is noted to be "sandwiched" between two closely spaced QRS complexes, the first of which originates from an ectopic focus (commonly, the A-V junction). As a result, the QRS complex following the retrograde P wave appears earlier than the usual R-R cycle of the basic rhythm. The R-R interval which includes the "sandwiched" P wave is usually 0.50 second or less. However, it may be slightly longer than 0.50 second when there is a marked conduction delay in retrograde and/or antegrade conduction.

The fundamental mechanism responsible for the genesis of reciprocal beats is considered to be a specific form of re-entry phenomenon occurring in the A-V junctional tissue. One assumes that there is a longitudinal dissociation present in the A-V junctional fibers, which have different degrees of depressed conductivity. Thus, some of the longitudinal fibers are more markedly depressed than others. Consequently, unidirectional block of retrograde conduction occurs in the more depressed fibers in addition to a generalized delay in retrograde conduction in the remaining fibers. The impulse originating from the A-V node is conducted in both directions, i.e., to the ventricles (antegrade) and toward the atria (retrograde). The retrograde impulse reaches the depressed A-V junctional fibers and is completely blocked in the more depressed fibers, while it is conducted at a slower speed than usual in a retrograde fashion in the remaining, less depressed fibers. The R-P interval in a reciprocal beat is consequently prolonged (longer than 0.20 second) because of the delayed retrograde conduction. In the meantime the more depressed longitudinal fibers, which were previously refractory to the retrograde impulse, recover their conductivity. As a result, the retrograde impulse splits before reaching the atria; one impulse continues in retrograde direction to the atria and another retraces its steps in antegrade direction toward the A-V node. In other words, the antegrade impulse traverses down the longitudinal fibers which are now responsive, but were previously refractory. When the time required (the R-R interval which includes the "sandwiched" P wave) for the retrograde conduction of the nodal impulse (R-P interval) and the subsequent antegrade conduction of the re-entry impulse (P-R interval) is sufficient for the ventricles to recover from their initial response to the nodal impulse, a second ventricular complex, namely, *the reciprocal beat*, will result.

The underlying cause to produce this arrhythmia was found to be digitalis intoxication (see Chapter 7).

Case 180

This ECG tracing was obtained from a 60-year-old woman with no demonstrable heart disease. She was not taking any drug.

What is your cardiac rhythm diagnosis?

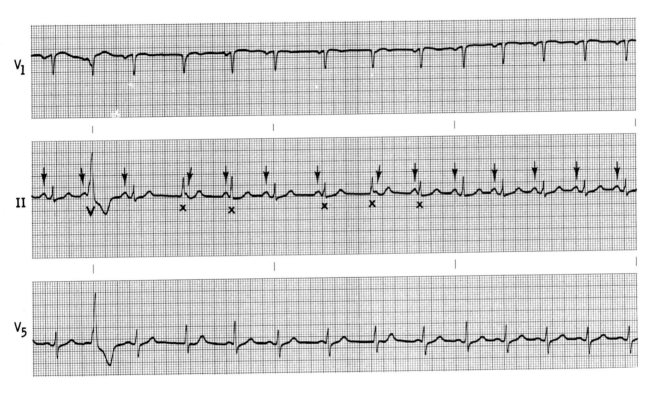

Case 180: Diagnosis

Arrows indicate sinus P waves. It should be noted that the P-P cycle changes from time to time in otherwise a regular rhythm. In other words, the longer P-P interval (cycle) is shorter than two basic P-P intervals. This ECG finding most likely represents Wenckebach sino-atrial (S-A) block. When the atrial rate is reduced during S-A block, A-V junctional escape beats (marked X) occur with slightly accelerated rate (the escape rate: 75 beats per minute), leading to incomplete A-V dissociation.

It should be noted that the configuration of the escape beats is slightly different from that of the basic sinus beats. This finding indicates that the escape beats may be arising from one of the fasicles of the left bundle branch system (see Cases 86, 107, and 108). Note a ventricular premature contraction (marked V).

Case 181

A 66-year-old man with a previous heart attack was examined at the cardiac clinic for the evaluation of his new cardiac arrhythmia. He was not taking any medication.

1. *What is your cardiac rhythm diagnosis?*
2. *What is most likely the underlying disorder responsible for the production of this arrhythmia?*

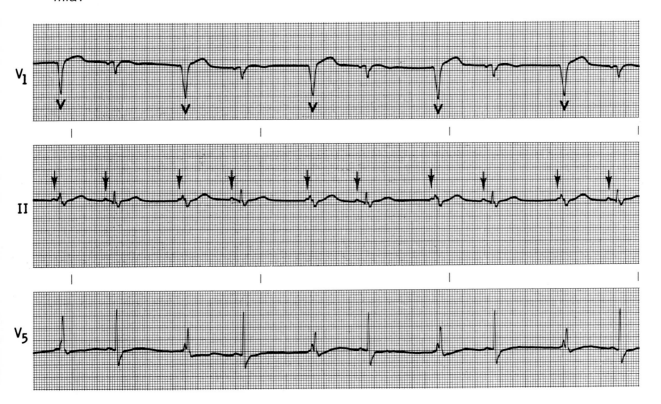

V₁

II

V₅

Case 181: Diagnosis

Arrows indicate sinus P waves. It is interesting to note that the P-P cycle reveals a regular irregularity—alternating short and long P-P intervals. The long P-P interval is shorter than two short P-P intervals indicating 3:2 Wenckebach S-A block (see Case 37).

Whenever the ventricular pause occurs as a result of S-A block, ventricular escape beats (marked V) appear to take over the ventricular activity. The term "ventricular escape-bigeminy" can be applied to explain this arrhythmia because the ventricular escape beats appear alternately with the sinus beats as a bigeminal form.

In this ECG tracing, the appearance of the ventricular escape beats in place of the expected A-V junctional escape beats most likely represents diseased A-V node.

As far as the underlying disorder to produce the above-mentioned electrophysiologic events is concerned, sick sinus syndrome (SSS) is most likely the diagnosis in view of the fact that S-A block is often due to diseased sinus node and also the diseased A-V node commonly coexists with SSS (see Chapter 1 and Case 1).

Case 182

A complex cardiac arrhythmia was observed on an 86-year-old man with a previous diaphragmatic lateral myocardial infarction. He had been taking a maintenance digoxin 0.125 mg. daily.

1. *What is your cardiac rhythm diagnosis?*
2. *What is the most likely cause in producing this arrhythmia?*

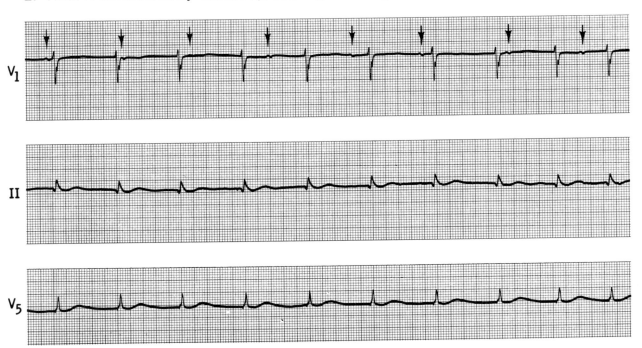

Case 182: Diagnosis

Arrows indicate P waves. The P-P cycle is irregular and the ventricular cycle is also irregular, but there is no relationship between the atrial and the ventricular activity. As far as the atrial activity is concerned, intermittent 3:2 sino-atrial (S-A) block is most likely the diagnosis (see Case 181). The ventricular activity is controlled by the A-V junctional focus with a rate of 62–65 beats per minute. In some areas (the last 4 beats), the R-R intervals progressively shorten and this finding most likely represents Wenckebach exit block. Thus, a complete cardiac rhythm diagnosis is sinus arrhythmia with intermittent 3:2 Wenckebach S-A block and independent nonparoxysmal A-V junctional tachycardia with intermittent Wenckebach exit block producing complete A-V dissociation. It is not uncommon to observe unclear and ill defined P waves with low amplitude in elderly people.

The underlying cause of this complex cardiac arrhythmia is either digitalis toxicity or SSS (see Chapters 1 and 7).

Case 183

These cardiac rhythm strips represent the Holter monitor ECG, and they are not continuous.

What is your cardiac rhythm diagnosis?

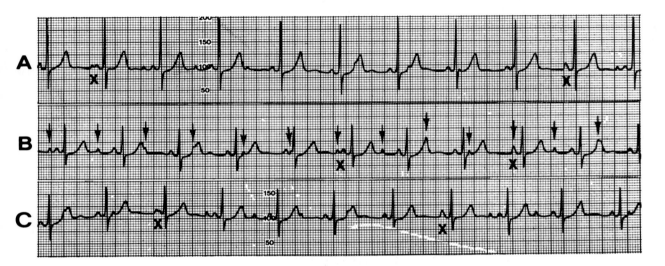

Case 183: Diagnosis

The underlying cardiac rhythm is sinus with a rate of 70 beats per minute, but there is another set of P waves (indicated by arrows). None of the ectopic P waves (indicated by arrows) are conducted to the ventricles, indicating unilateral atrial rhythm with a rate of 83 beats per minute. Thus, the cardiac rhythm diagnosis is atrial dissociation. Note that some P waves are tall and deformed (marked X) when the sinus P waves and the ectopic P waves occur simultaneously.

It is extremely important to emphasize that the extra P waves causing unilateral atrial rhythm may actually be due to artifacts. Thus, a possibility of artifacts must be always considered when dealing with atrial dissociation.

Case 184

This ECG tracing was taken on a 61-year-old woman with mild hypertension. She was not taking any medication.

What is your ECG diagnosis?

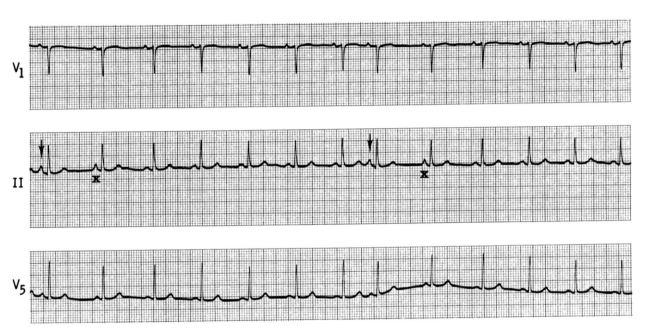

Case 184: Diagnosis

The underlying cardiac rhythm is sinus with a rate of 78 beats per minute. There are two APCs (indicated by arrows) followed by bizzare P waves (marked X) of the sinus beats. The bizarre P wave of the sinus beat immediately following any ectopic beat (commonly APC) is termed "aberrant atrial conduction" or "Chung's phenomenon." Chung's phenomenon is considered to be due to alteration of the refractoriness in the atria soon after any ectopic beat. The aberrant atrial conduction usually involves only one sinus beat following any ectopic beat, but it may involve two or more sinus P waves consecutively.

Chung's phenomenon is not uncommon in elderly people, but the finding is nonspecific, with no clinical significance.

chapter 10

Miscellaneous

Case 185

A 67-year-old woman developed a life-threatening cardiac arrhythmia while she was taking a cardiac drug. Leads II-a, b, c, and d are continuous.

1. *What is your cardiac rhythm diagnosis?*
2. *What cardiac drug is most likely responsible for the production of this arrhythmia?*

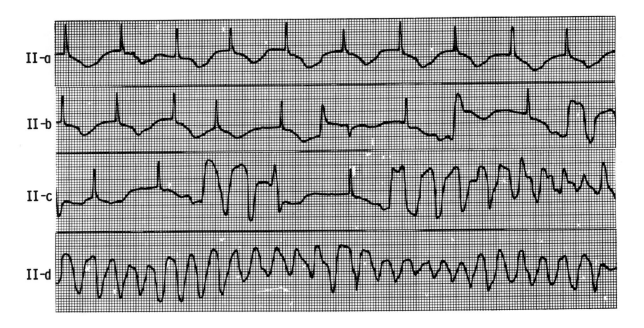

Case 185: Diagnosis

The atrial activity is not clearly evident. The basic cardiac rhythm, therefore, is most likely atrial fibrillation with predominantly nonparoxysmal A-V junctional tachycardia (rate: 72 beats per minute). Multiformed ventricular tachycardia (VT) (rate: 180–215 beats per minute) is produced by ventricular premature contractions (VPCs) with the R-on-T phenomenon as a result of markedly prolonged Q-T interval with broad T wave due to quinidine, and it is deteriorated to ventricular fibrillation. This type of irregular and multiformed VT is termed "torsades de pointes."

In 1966, Dessertenne had applied the term "torsades de pointes" to describe paroxysmal VT (usually faster than 180–200 beats per minute) with multiple configurations of the QRS complexes and prefibrillatory patterns so that the entire QRS complexes appear to be twisting about the baseline. The original meaning of "torsades de pointes" is "twisting of the points."

Torsades de pointes type of VT has been reported to be commonly associated with a prolonged Q-T interval usually due to quinidine or a similar antiarrhythmic drug (e.g., Pronestyl, Norpace, etc.). In addition, this arrhythmia may be initiated by the prolonged Q-T interval due to other drugs such as prenylamine, phenothiazines, and amitryptiline. Furthermore, hypokalemia-induced torsades de pointes has been reported in the literature.

Since torsades de pointes is considered to be a precursor to ventricular fibrillation and sudden death, the causative drug to prolong the Q-T interval must be discontinued immediately, and the patient has to be closely monitored. Direct current shock and various resuscitative measures must be applied without delay as needed.

Case 186

A 19-year-old man in a semiunconscious state was brought to the emergency room by a police officer following an automobile accident which took place on a very cold day. It was uncertain how long he had been exposed to the cold air before the officer discovered him.

1. *What is your ECG diagnosis?*
2. *What is the usual cause of this ECG abnormality?*

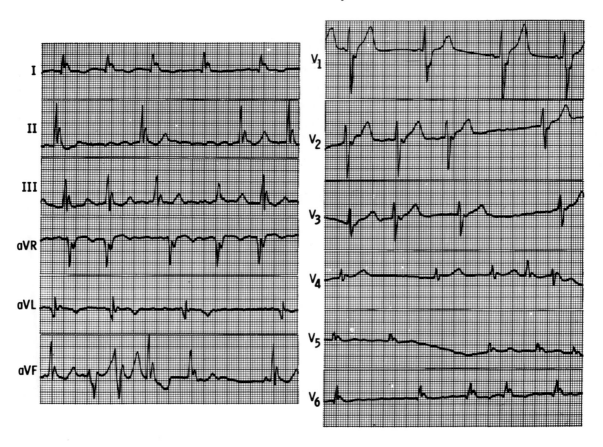

Case 186: Diagnosis

The underlying rhythm is a very unstable sinus bradycardia and intermittent atrial flutter-fibrillation with advanced A-V block producing a slow ventricular rate (rate: 40–60 beats per minute).

All QRS complexes of this ECG tracing are bizarre and broad, indicating diffuse (nonspecific) intraventricular block. This ECG abnormality is often produced by hypothermia—exposure to the cold air for unknown duration. In addition, the R wave is tall in lead V_1, and there are significant Q waves in leads I, aVL, and V_6 suggestive of posterolateral myocardial infarction (MI). MI is not uncommon following an automobile accident when the heart, including coronary artery(ies), is (are) injured by a steering wheel. Of course, a sudden exposure to the very cold air itself may cause acute coronary artery spasm leading to MI.

Markedly unstable sinus bradycardia with intermittent atrial flutter-fibrillation with advanced A-V block represents sick sinus syndrome (see Chapter 1) directly due to hypothermia. In lead aVF, some QRS complexes are even more bizarre than the remaining beats. This ECG finding is most likely due to aberrant ventricular conduction.

In summary, the above-mentioned ECG abnormalities are directly the end result of hypothermia following an automobile accident on a cold day, although the steering wheel injury may be responsible for the production of MI. Unfortunately, all available resuscitative measures were unsuccessful. Autopsy permission was not granted.

Case 187

A 46-year-old man was referred to a cardiologist for evaluation of chest pain. He was not taking any drugs. His physical findings were negative and his 12-lead ECG was within normal limits (not shown here).

He was unable to continue the exercise testing beyond stage 2 of the exercise protocol because of frequent ventricular premature contractions (VPCs) associated with a significant S-T segment depression. His maximal heart rate was only 103 beats per minute. A single channel (modified lead V_5) was utilized.

1. *What is the exercise ECG diagnosis?*
2. *What is its clinical significance?*

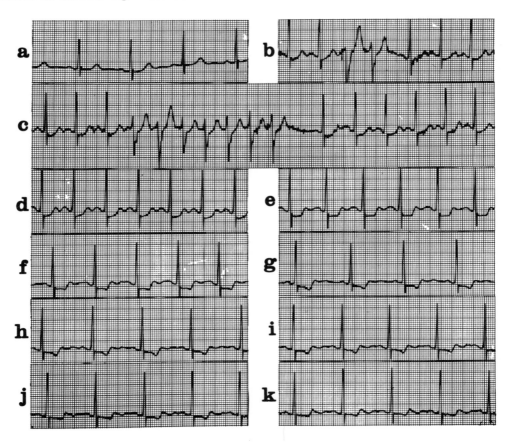

Case 187: Diagnosis

Strip A is a resting tracing; strip B was recorded during exercise. The remaining strips, C through K, are postexercise tracings.

The patient developed frequent VPCs with paroxysmal ventricular tachycardia (VT) soon after the initiation of exercise; these were associated with a significant horizontal to downsloping S-T segment depression. It has been well documented that ventricular arrhythmias, particularly multifocal VPCs, grouped VPCs, and VT provoked by minimal exercise (with less than 70% of the predicted maximal heart rate) are highly suggestive of significant coronary artery disease. The exercise ECG test was, of course, markedly positive.

Case 188

The ECG tracing shown in this page (tracing, A) was taken with the usual ECG electrode placement, whereas another ECG tracing (tracing, B) shown in the next page was recorded by reversing the left and the right arm electrode placement with the right precordial leads (the chest leads were taken by placing the electrodes exactly on the opposite sites of the conventional leads V_{1-6}) on a 66-year-old man with mild hypertension.

What is your ECG diagnosis?

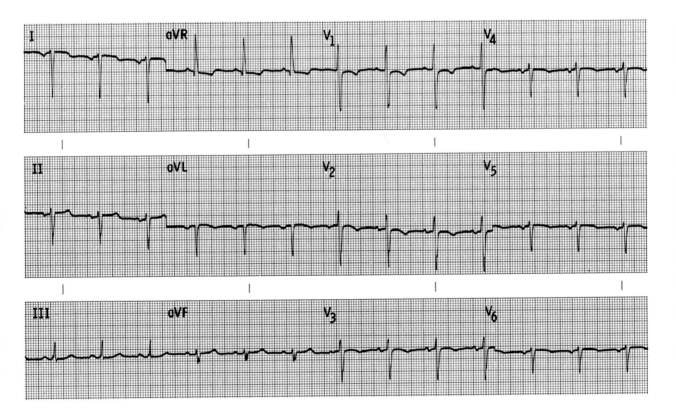

Case 188: Diagnosis

The cardiac rhythm is sinus with a rate of 78 beats per minute. The *tracing A* (conventional lead placement) reveals a very unusual ECG pattern because of a mirror-image dextrocardia. Note that the entire ECG complexes are inversed (downward) in lead I, and lead aVL looks like the usual lead aVR in tracing A. The amplitude of the R waves progressively reduced in the precordial leads rather than the usual progressive increment of the R wave amplitude in tracing A.

The *tracing B* taken with the reversed electrode placement between the left and the right arm and the right precordial leads reveal the usual ECG pattern.

Left ventricular hypertrophy and anteroseptal myocardial ischemia are suggested.

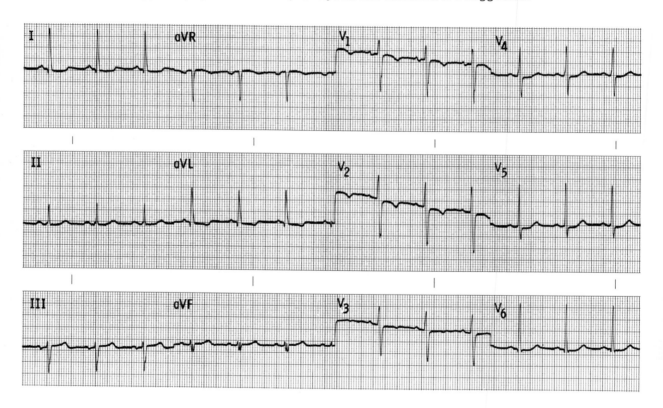

Cardiac consultation was requested on a 27-year-old man for the evaluation of a heart murmur along with an abnormal ECG finding and atypical chest pain.

1. *What is your ECG diagnosis?*
1. *What is the best therapeutic approach?*

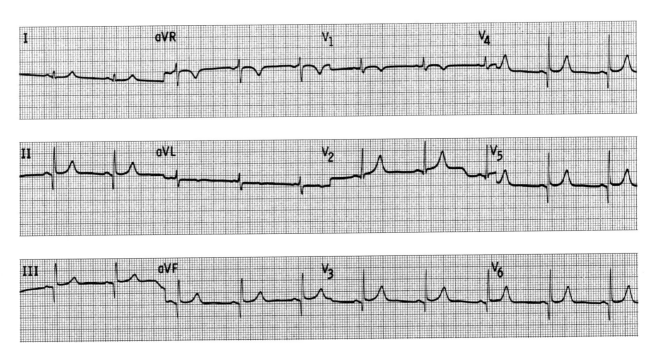

Case 189: Diagnosis

The cardiac rhythm is sinus bradycardia with a rate of 57 beats per minute. The P-R interval is relatively short, but there is no evidence of Wolff-Parkinson-White syndrome (see Chapter 6).

The striking ECG abnormalities include deep but narrow Q waves in leads II, III, aVF, and V_{3-6} with a relatively tall R wave in lead V_1, suggestive of old diaphragmatic posterolateral MI. This ECG finding is actually due to ventricular septal hypertrophy as a result of idiopathic hypertrophic subaortic stenosis (IHSS). It should be noted that IHSS frequently causes *pseudo* MI pattern by virtue of the ventricular septal hypertrophy. As a rule, the Q waves are deep but narrow in inferior leads and/or the left precordial leads and T waves are usually upright in IHSS.

Beta blocking agents (e.g., propranolol) are often effective to relieve various symptoms in IHSS, but the surgical approach is occasionally indicated for advanced cases.

Case 190

A 26-year-old man who has been healthy during his entire life was brought to the emergency room because of a sharp chest pain with a few hours in duration. He gave a history of ''flu-like'' symptoms prior to the development of chest pain.

What is your ECG diagnosis?

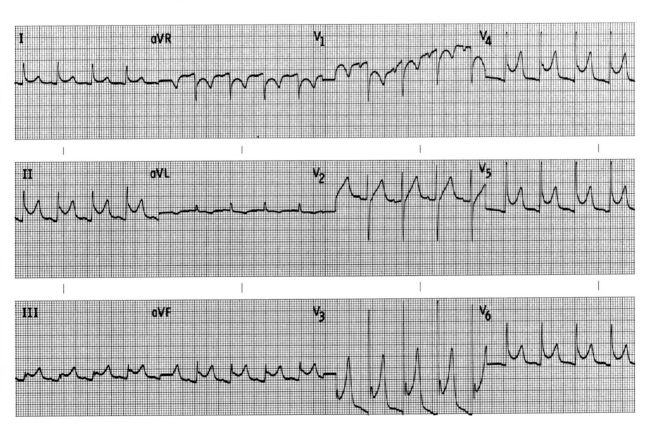

Case 190: Diagnosis

The cardiac rhythm is sinus tachycardia with a rate of 103 beats per minute. It is easy to recognize marked S-T segment elevation involving diffusely many leads. This finding is the characteristic ECG abnormality seen in acute pericarditis.

During the early phase of acute pericarditis, upward concave elevation of the S-T segment occurs diffusely in practically all leads except lead aVR (and sometimes lead V_1). Because of the diffuse process in pericarditis, no reciprocal depression of the S-T segment is observed. Remember that acute MI characteristically produces a reciprocal S-T segment depression in the ECG leads facing the uninvolved myocardium during the first 72 hours.

During the late stage (e.g., the subacute and chronic phases) of pericarditis, the S-T segment elevation returns to the isoelectric line, but the T waves begin to be inverted in many leads. The T wave inversion in pericarditis may last for weeks or months. It is extremely important to remember that abnormal Q waves never occur in uncomplicated pericarditis.

This patient was found to have acute viral pericarditis.

Case 191

This ECG tracing was recorded on a 29-year-old man a few hours following surgical repair for atrial septal defect. He was not taking any medication.

1. *What is your ECG diagnosis?*
2. *What is the treatment of choice?*

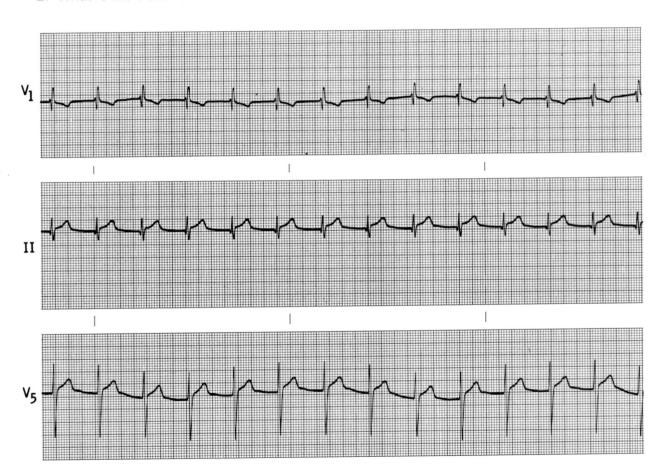

Case 191: Diagnosis

The cardiac rhythm is nonparoxysmal A-V junctional tachycardia with a rate of 87 beats per minute. Note that the ventricular cycle is precisely regular but there is no P wave.

There is S-T segment elevation involving diffusely many leads (only 3 leads are shown here) indicative of acute pericarditis. The term "postpericardiotomy syndrome" or "postcardiotomy syndrome" is commonly used to designate acute pericarditis resulting from any form of trauma (including surgical trauma) to the heart.

In atrial septal defect, right bundle branch block (RBBB) pattern (either complete or incomplete) is very common (up to 90% of cases).

Nonparoxysmal A-V junctional tachycardia is a relatively common cardiac arrhythmia following various cardiac operations, but it is usually self-limited. Thus, no treatment is indicated. Likewise, no treatment is necessary for the postcardiotomy syndrome unless the patient suffers from significant symptoms (e.g., chest pain, fever, etc.) due to the surgery-induced pericarditis.

Case 192

A 54-year-old man who had recovered from a heart attack 6 months previously developed a new cardiac arrhythmia soon after coronary artery bypass surgery. He was not taking any drug except for aspirin 2 tablets daily.

1. *What is your cardiac rhythm diagnosis?*
2. *What is the proper management for this arrhythmia?*
3. *What is the location of a previous heart attack?*

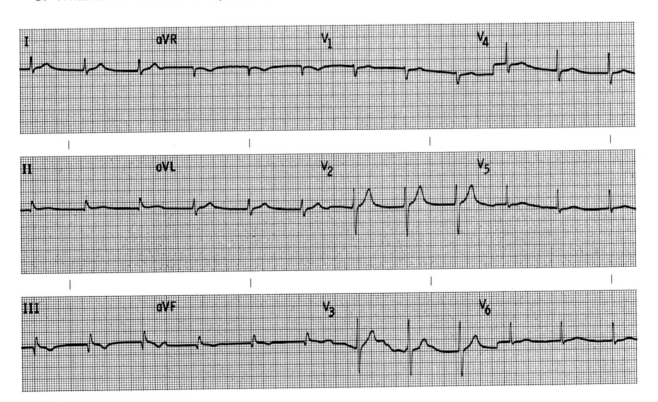

Case 192: Diagnosis

The cardiac rhythm diagnosis is nonparoxysmal A-V junctional tachycardia with a rate of 72 beats per minute. The R-R intervals are regular throughout the tracing without discernible P wave. When there is no P wave under this circumstance, the finding usually indicates that the atria and the ventricles are activated simultaneously so that the retrograde P wave is superimposed on the QRS complex in each cycle rather than assuming atrial standstill.

As indicated earlier (see Case 191), nonparoxysmal A-V junctional tachycardia is not uncommon following various cardiac surgeries including coronary artery bypass surgery. No treatment is indicated for this arrhythmia.

It is easy to recognize evidence of old diaphragmatic MI (Q waves in leads II, III, and aVF). In addition, postcardiotomy syndrome is suggested on the basis of a slight S-T segment elevation in many leads (see Cases 190 and 191).

Case 193

A 60-year-old woman with a long-standing renal failure had expired soon after this ECG tracing was recorded.

1. *What is your ECG diagnosis?*
2. *What electrolyte imbalance(s) is (are) present?*

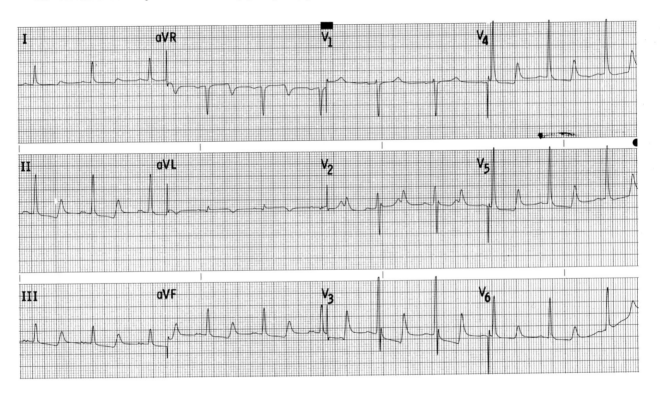

Case 193: Diagnosis

The cardiac rhythm is sinus with a rate of 64 beats per minute. There are two striking ECG abnormalities including tall and peaked T wave and markedly prolonged Q-T interval.

The tall and peaked T wave with narrow base is a characteristic ECG abnormality of hyperkalemia. When hyperkalemia further advances, the above-mentioned ECG finding is followed by flat P wave (at times no P wave at all), first degree A-V block and various intraventricular blocks. In terminal cases of far advanced hyperkalemia, the cardiac rhythm eventually will deteriorate to VT and fibrillation leading to idioventricular rhythm and ventricular standstill.

Another striking ECG abnormality is markedly prolonged Q-T interval, which is a typical manifestation of hypocalcemia. The primary reason for the prolongation of the Q-T interval in hypocalcemia is the lengthening of the S-T segment. The T wave itself is *not* altered either by hypocalcemia or hypercalcemia.

It is rather common to observe a combination of hyperkalemia and hypocalcemia in patients with advanced renal failure.

The diagnosis of left ventricular hypertrophy can be readily made, and left atrial enlargement is also suggested. The amplitude of the P wave is relatively low because of hyperkalemia.

Case 194

This ECG tracing was obtained from a 62-year-old woman with breast cancer.

1. *What is your ECG diagnosis?*
2. *What electrolyte imbalance is responsible for the production of this ECG abnormality?*

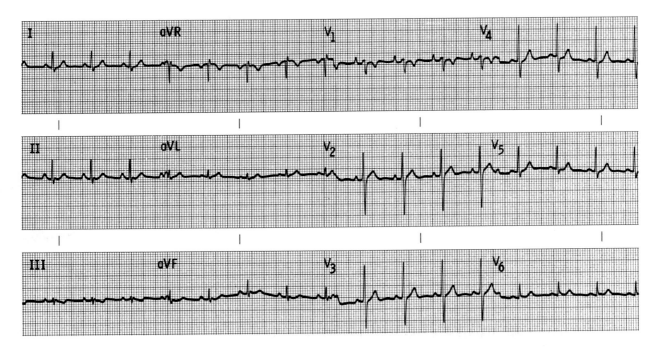

Case 194: Diagnosis

The cardiac rhythm is sinus with a rate of 94 beats per minute. The striking ECG abnormality in this tracing is a very short Q-T interval (0.26 second) due to hypercalcemia. The short Q-T interval in hypercalcemia is directly due to a shortening of or a virtual disappearance of the S-T segment. The T wave itself is *not* altered by hypercalcemia, however.

This patient was found to have diffuse metastasis to the bones arising from her breast cancer.

Case 195

This ECG tracing was taken on a 34-year-old woman. She was not taking any medication.

1. *What is your ECG diagnosis?*
2. *What are the common causes of prolonged Q-T interval?*

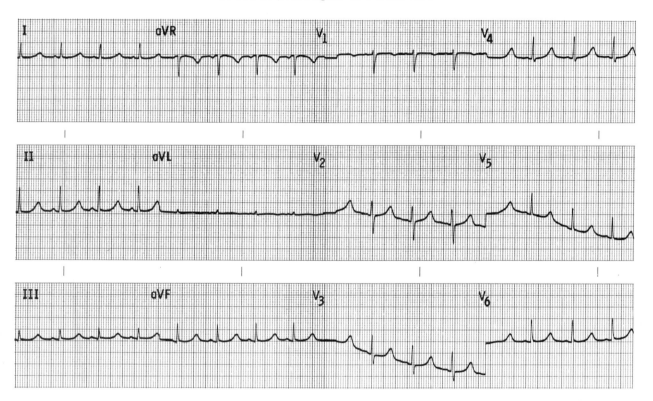

Case 195: Diagnosis

The cardiac rhythm is sinus with a rate of 90 beats per minute. It is easy to recognize that the Q-T interval is significantly prolonged as a result of hypocalcemia (the Q-T interval: 0.40 second). As described previously, the prolonged Q-T interval in hypocalcemia is due to the lengthening of the S-T segment (see Case 193). This patient was referred to the endocrinology clinic for further evaluation of hypocalcemia. Common causes of the Q-T interval prolongation may include:

Hypocalcemia

Quinidine (or similar anti-arrhythmic drugs such as procainamide) effect (see Cases 144 and 185)

Various drugs (e.g., antidepressants, tranquilizers) used for mental disorders

Central nervous system disorders (see Case 196)

Acute coronary event (e.g., myocardial ischemia, acute MI)

Hypothermia (see Case 186)

Old age, and

Congenital Q-T syndrome (congenital prolongation of the Q-T interval with or without deafness associated with high incidence of sudden death).

Case 196

A 63-year-old woman was admitted to the neurology service for the evaluation and management of a stroke. She was not taking any medication.

What is your ECG diagnosis?

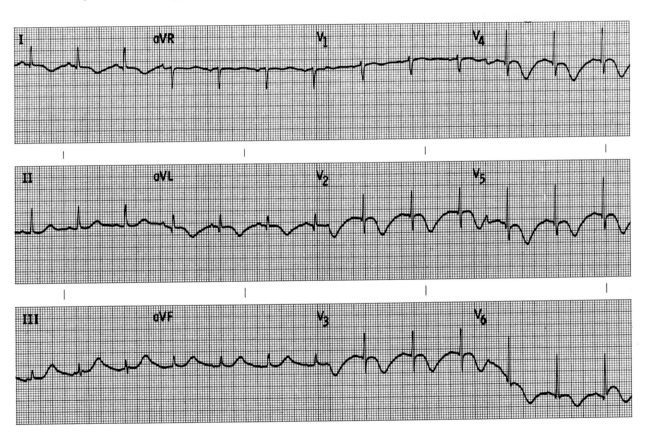

Case 196: Diagnosis

The cardiac rhythm is sinus with a rate of 75 beats per minute. The Q-T interval is markedly prolonged as a result of broad T waves, and the T waves are inverted in many leads. These ECG findings are relatively common in a variety of central nervous system disorders. Subarachnoid hemorrhage is probably the most common disorder to produce the above findings.

The exact underlying mechanism responsible for the production of the Q-T interval prolongation in central nervous system disorders is not fully understood. Myocardial ischemia does not seem to be responsible for the production of this phenomenon. The prolongation of the Q-T interval in central nervous system disorders may or may not be associated with inverted T waves.

In addition to the primary central nervous system disorders, the Q-T interval is often prolonged when any individual suffers from hepatic coma, diabetic coma, advanced renal failure, delirium tremens, and cardiac arrest from a variety of causes. The Q-T interval may return to a normal value when the underlying disorders responsible for the production of the Q-T interval prolongation are well controlled or cured.

Case 197

A 12-year-old girl was seen at the pediatric clinic during an annual check-up.

What is your ECG diagnosis?

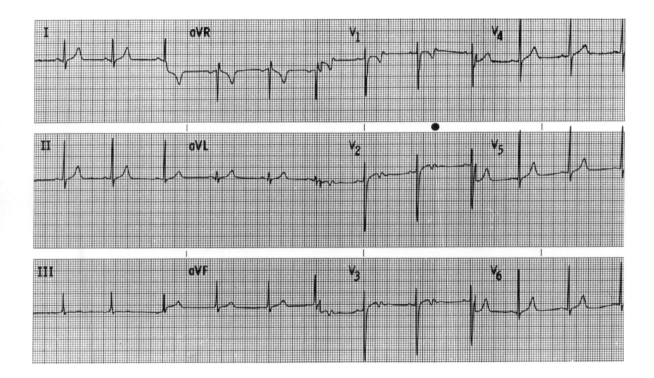

Case 197: Diagnosis

The cardiac rhythm is sinus arrhythmia with a rate of 70 beats per minute. It is interesting to note that the T waves are biphasic and irregular in shape in leads V_1 through V_3. This ECG finding is a good example of the juvenile T wave pattern.

In most cases, the T waves are inverted (not deeply or symmetrically) in leads V_1 through V_3 (at times up to leads V_4 through V_6) in the juvenile T wave pattern, but occasionally the T wave configuration may show a biphasic or irregular pattern.

This girl was found to be perfectly healthy, and the ECG finding was also within normal limits.

Case 198

A 47-year-old woman was brought to the emergency room because she developed a sharp pain in the chest associated with severe dyspnea of a few hours in duration.

1. *What is your ECG diagnosis?*
2. *What is the underlying disorder responsible for the production of these ECG abnormalities?*
3. *What other ECG findings may be produced by this clinical entity?*

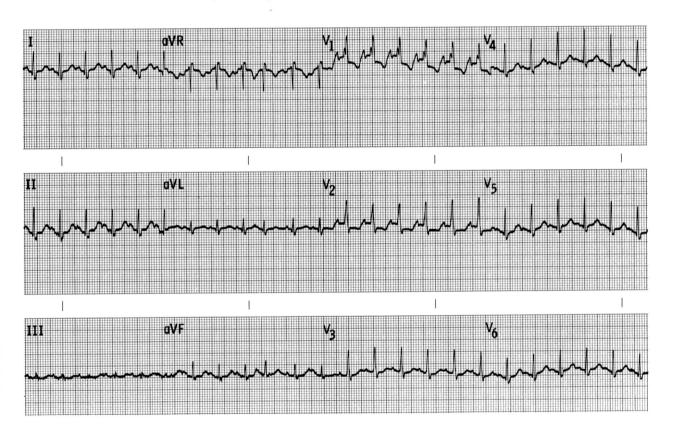

Case 198: Diagnosis

The underlying cardiac rhythm is marked sinus tachycardia with a rate of 140 beats per minute. Note occasional atrial premature contractions (APC). There are two striking ECG abnormalities including RBBB and P-pulmonale. These ECG findings are typically due to acute pulmonary embolism.

Common ECG abnormalities in pulmonary embolism may include:

Marked sinus tachycardia

Righ axis deviation (new onset)

RBBB (complete or incomplete) of new onset

P-pulmonale

Acute atrial tachyarrhythmias (e.g., frequent APCs, atrial tachycardia, atrial fibrillation, atrial flutter, and multifocal atrial tachycardia)

Inverted T waves in leads V_{1-3} (acute right ventricular strain pattern)

Inverted T waves in leads II, III and aVF

Posterior axis deviation (former term, "clockwise rotation")

S_1-Q_3 pattern (deep S wave in lead I and deep Q wave in lead III)

Pseudo-diaphragmatic MI pattern, and

$S_1-S_2-S_3$ pattern (deep S waves in leads I, II, and III)

On rare occasions, pulmonary embolism may cause marked left axis deviation.

Case 199

This ECG tracing was obtained from a 52-year-old man with coronary artery disease. He was not taking any medication except for occasional use of sublingual nitroglycerin.

What is your cardiac rhythm diagnosis?

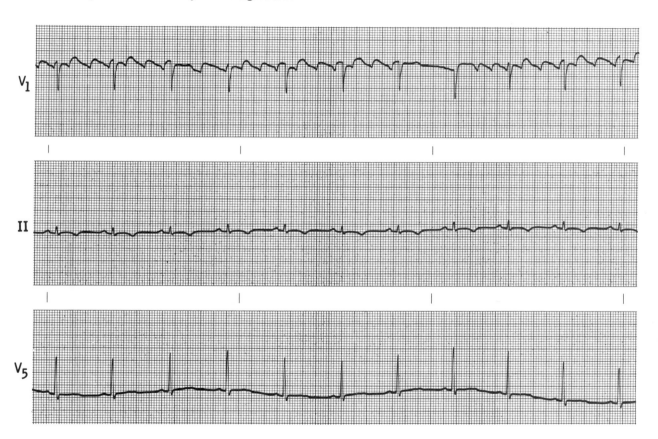

Case 199: Diagnosis

The underlying cardiac rhythm is sinus with a rate of 70 beats per minute, but lead V_1 appears to show atrial flutter. This *pseudo*-atrial flutter *pattern* represents artifacts which are due to partially broken down electrode wire of lead V_1 connected to the ECG machine. Remember that leads V_1, II and V_5 are taken simultaneously using 3-channel ECG recorder. Therefore, it is impossible to have atrial flutter or any other cardiac arrhythmias in lead V_1 while other ECG leads (II and V_5) reveal normal sinus rhythm.

It is extremely important to consider a possibility of various artifacts when dealing with any complex cardiac arrhythmias or any unexplainable cardiac rhythm disturbances.

Case 200

Cardiac consultation was requested on a 55-year-old man with no demonstrable heart disease because of unusual ECG findings which appear to be a complex cardiac arrhythmia.

What is your cardiac rhythm diagnosis?

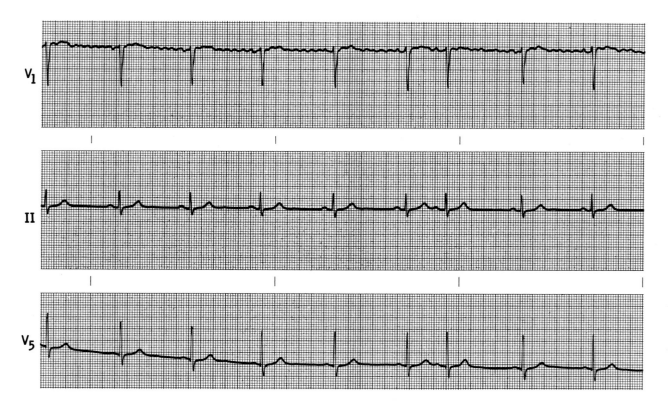

441

Case 200: Diagnosis

The underlying cardiac rhythm is sinus bradycardia with a rate of 52 beats per minute and there is an APC (the 7th beat). Lead V_1 appears to show atrial fibrillation because of artifacts due to improper contact of the ECG electrode with the skin surface of that lead. As stressed previously, it is impossible to expect any type of cardiac arrhythmia in any given ECG lead during sinus rhythm which is evident in the remaining ECG leads when multiple ECG leads are recorded simultaneously.

Remember that various artifacts may resemble almost every kind of cardiac arrhythmia. Unless the ECG reader is fully familiar with various artifacts, an erroneous ECG interpretation may not be avoided, so that unnecessary and even harmful management may be provided.

Suggested Readings

1. Chung, E.K.: *Quick Reference to Cardiovascular Diseases*, Second Edition, Philadelphia, Lippincott/Harper & Row, 1982.
2. Chung, E.K.: *Ambulatory Electrocardiography: Holter Monitor Electrocardiography*, New York, Springer-Verlag, 1980.
3. Chung, E.K.: *Cardiac Emergency Care*, Second Edition, Philadelphia, Lea & Febiger, 1980.
4. Chung, E.K.: *Electrocardiography: Practical Applications with Vectorial Principles*, Second Edition, Hagerstown, Md., Harper & Row, 1980.
5. Chung, E.K.: Sick sinus syndrome: Current views (part I). *Mod. Conc. Cardiovasc. Dis. 49:*61, 1980.
6. Chung, E.K.: Sick sinus syndrome: Current views (part II). *Mod. Conc. Cardiovasc. Dis. 49:*67, 1980.
7. Chung, E.K.: *Artificial Cardiac Pacing: Practical Approach*, Baltimore, Williams & Wilkins, 1979.
8. Chung, E.K.: *Exercise Electrocardiography: Practical Approach*, Baltimore, Williams & Wilkins, 1979.
9. Chung, E.K.: *Cardiac Arrhythmias: Self Assessment, Volume - I*, Baltimore, Williams & Wilkins, 1977.
10. Chung, E.K.: *Principles of Cardiac Arrhythmias*, Second Edition, Baltimore, Williams & Wilkins, 1977.
11. Chung, E.K.: Wolff-Parkinson-White syndrome: Current views. *Am. J. Med. 62:*252, 1977.
12. Chung, E.K.: *Digitalis Intoxication*, Amsterdam, Netherlands, Excerpta Medica (Baltimore, Williams & Wilkins), 1969.
13. Dhingra, R.C., Wyndham, C., Bauernfeind, R., et al.: Significance of chronic bifascicular block without apparent organic heart disease. *Circulation 60:*33, 1979.
14. Doherty, J.E., Straub, K.D., Murphy, M.L., et al.: Digoxin-quinidine interaction: Changes in canine tissue concentration from steady state with quinidine. *Am. J. Cardiol. 45:*1196, 1980.
15. Fenster, P.E., Powell, J.R., Graves, P.E., et al.: Digitoxin-quinidine interaction: Pharmacokinetic evaluation. *Ann. Intern. Med. 93:*5, 1980.
16. Fisch, G.R., Zipes, D.P., Fisch, C.: Bundle branch block and sudden death. *Prog. Cardiovasc. Dis. 23:*187, 1980.
17. Garty, M., Sood, P., Rollins, D.E.: Digitoxin elimination reduced during quinidine therapy. *Ann. Intern. Med. 94:*1, 1981.
18. Gold, F.L., From, A.H.L.: Alternating bundle branch block. *J. Electrocard. 13:*405, 1980.
19. Horowitz, L.N., Greenspan, A.M., Spielman, S.R., Josephson, M.E.: Torsades de pointes: Electrophysiologic studies in patients without transient pharmacologic or metabolic abnormalities. *Circulation 63:*1120, 1981.
20. Josephson, M.E., and Seides, S.F.: *Clinical Cardiac Electrophysiology: Techniques and Interpretations*, Philadelphia, Lea & Febiger, 1979.
21. Kostis, J.B., McCrone, K., Moreyra, A.E., et al.: Premature ventricular complexes in the absence of identifiable heart disease. *Circulation 63:*1351, 1981.
22. Levy, S., Roudaut, R., Bouvier, E., et al.: Alternate ventriculoatrial Wenckebach conduction. *Circulation 61:*648, 1980.
23. Lewis, S., Kanakis, C., Rosen, K.M., Denes, P.: Significance of site of origin of premature ventricular contractions. *Am. Heart J. 97:*159, 1979.
24. Lyons, C.: Site of functional right bundle branch block. *Am. Heart J. 100:*653, 1980.
25. Marriott, H.J.L.: *Practical Electrocardiography*, Sixth Edition, Baltimore, Williams & Wilkins, 1977.
26. Moss, A.J.: Clinical significance of ventricular arrhythmias in patients with and without coronary artery disease. *Prog. Cardiovas. Dis. 23:*33, 1980.
27. Mungall, D.R., Robichaux, R.P., Perry, W., et al.: Effects of quinidine on serum digoxin concentration: A prospective study. *Ann. Intern. Med. 93:*5, 1980.
28. Narula, O.S.: *Cardiac Arrhythmias: Electrophysiology, Diagnosis and Management*, Baltimore, Williams & Wilkins, 1979.
29. Papa, L., Saia, J.A., and Chung, E.K.: Ventricular fibrillation in Wolff-Parkinson-White syndrome, type A. *Heart and Lung 7(6):*1015, 1978.
30. Perloff, J.K., Roberts, N.K., Cabeen, W.R.: Left axis deviation: A reassessment. *Circulation 60:*12, 1979.
31. Schamroth, L.: *The Disorders of Cardiac Rhythm*, Second Edition, Oxford, Blackwell Scientific Pub., 1980.
32. Schamroth, L.: Ventricular extrasystoles, ventricular tachycardia, and ventricular fibrillation: clinical electrocardiographic considerations. *Prog. Cardiovas. Dis. 23:*13, 1980.
33. Schneider, J.F., Thomas, H.E., Jr., Sorlie, P., et al.: Comparative features of newly acquired left and right bundle branch block in the general population: the Framingham study. *Am. J. Cardiol. 47:*931, 1981.
34. Schneider, J.F., Thomas, H.E., Jr., Kreger, B.E., et al.: Newly acquired right bundle-branch block: The Framingham study. *Ann. Intern. Med. 92:*37, 1980.
35. Sharma, P.R., and Chung, E.K.: Clinical implication of

surface morphology of ventricular premature contractions, *J. Electrocard. 13(4):*331, 1980.

36. Smith, W.M., Gallagher, J.J.: "Les Torsades de Pointes": an unusual ventricular arrhythmia. *Ann. Intern. Med. 93:*578, 1980.

37. Steinbrecher, U.P., Fitchett, D.H. torsade de pointes: a cause of syncope with atrioventricular block. *Arch. Intern. Med. 140:*1223, 1980.

38. Strasberg, M.D., Amat-Y-Leon, F., Dhingra, R.C., et al.: Natural history of chronic second-degree atrioventricular nodal block. *Circulation 63:*1043, 1981.

39. Tye, K.H., Samant, A., Dessler, K.B., Benchimol, A.: R on T or R on R phenomenon? Relation to the genesis of ventricular tachycardia. *Am. J. Cardiol. 44:*632, 1979.

40. Vetter, V.L., Josephson, M.E., Horowitz, L.N.: Idiopathic recurrent sustained ventricular tachycardia in children and adolescents. *Am. J. Cardiol. 47:*315, 1981.

41. Waldo, A.L., Wells, J.L., Jr., Cooper, T.B., MacLean, W.A.H.: Temporary cardiac pacing: applications and techniques in the treatment of cardiac arrhythmias. *Prog. Cardiovas. Dis. 23:*451, 1981.

42. Wellens, H.J.J., Bär, F.W.H.M., Lie, K.I.: The value of the electrocardiogram in the differential diagnosis of a tachycardia with a widened QRS complex. *Am. J. Med. 64:*27, 1978.

43. Zeppilli, P., Fenici, R., Sassara, M., et al.: Wenckebach second-degree A-V block in top-ranking athletes: an old problem revisited. *Am. Heart J. 100:*281, 1980.

Index*